MEDICATIONS IN SINGLE-DOSE VIALS

Implications of Discarded Drugs

AF622467

Edward H. Shortliffe, Francis K. Amankwah,
Tracy A. Lustig, and Sharyl J. Nass, *Editors*

Committee on Implications of Discarded Weight-Based Drugs

Board on Health Care Services

Health and Medicine Division

A Consensus Study Report of

The National Academies of
SCIENCES · ENGINEERING · MEDICINE

THE NATIONAL ACADEMIES PRESS
Washington, DC
www.nap.edu

THE NATIONAL ACADEMIES PRESS **500 Fifth Street, NW Washington, DC 20001**

This activity was supported by an agreement between the National Academy of Sciences and Centers for Medicare & Medicaid Services, U.S. Department of Health and Human Services. Any opinions, findings, conclusions, or recommendations expressed in this publication do not necessarily reflect the views of any organization or agency that provided support for the project.

International Standard Book Number-13: 978-0-309-68207-7
International Standard Book Number-10: 0-309-68207-X
Digital Object Identifier: https://doi.org/10.17226/25911
Library of Congress Control Number: 2021932057

Additional copies of this publication are available from the National Academies Press, 500 Fifth Street, NW, Keck 360, Washington, DC 20001; (800) 624-6242 or (202) 334-3313; http://www.nap.edu.

Copyright 2021 by the National Academy of Sciences. All rights reserved.

Printed in the United States of America

Suggested citation: National Academies of Sciences, Engineering, and Medicine. 2021. *Medications in single-dose vials: Implications of discarded drugs.* Washington, DC: The National Academies Press. https://doi.org/10.17226/25911.

The National Academies of

SCIENCES · ENGINEERING · MEDICINE

The **National Academy of Sciences** was established in 1863 by an Act of Congress, signed by President Lincoln, as a private, nongovernmental institution to advise the nation on issues related to science and technology. Members are elected by their peers for outstanding contributions to research. Dr. Marcia McNutt is president.

The **National Academy of Engineering** was established in 1964 under the charter of the National Academy of Sciences to bring the practices of engineering to advising the nation. Members are elected by their peers for extraordinary contributions to engineering. Dr. John L. Anderson is president.

The **National Academy of Medicine** (formerly the Institute of Medicine) was established in 1970 under the charter of the National Academy of Sciences to advise the nation on medical and health issues. Members are elected by their peers for distinguished contributions to medicine and health. Dr. Victor J. Dzau is president.

The three Academies work together as the **National Academies of Sciences, Engineering, and Medicine** to provide independent, objective analysis and advice to the nation and conduct other activities to solve complex problems and inform public policy decisions. The National Academies also encourage education and research, recognize outstanding contributions to knowledge, and increase public understanding in matters of science, engineering, and medicine.

Learn more about the National Academies of Sciences, Engineering, and Medicine at **www.nationalacademies.org**.

The National Academies of

SCIENCES · ENGINEERING · MEDICINE

Consensus Study Reports published by the National Academies of Sciences, Engineering, and Medicine document the evidence-based consensus on the study's statement of task by an authoring committee of experts. Reports typically include findings, conclusions, and recommendations based on information gathered by the committee and the committee's deliberations. Each report has been subjected to a rigorous and independent peer-review process and it represents the position of the National Academies on the statement of task.

Proceedings published by the National Academies of Sciences, Engineering, and Medicine chronicle the presentations and discussions at a workshop, symposium, or other event convened by the National Academies. The statements and opinions contained in proceedings are those of the participants and are not endorsed by other participants, the planning committee, or the National Academies.

For information about other products and activities of the National Academies, please visit www.nationalacademies.org/about/whatwedo.

COMMITTEE ON IMPLICATIONS OF DISCARDED WEIGHT-BASED DRUGS

EDWARD SHORTLIFFE (*Chair*), Chair Emeritus and Adjunct Professor of Biomedical Informatics, Columbia University; Adjunct Professor of Biomedical Informatics, Arizona State University; Adjunct Professor of Population Health Sciences, Weill Cornell Medical College

JULIE DONOHUE, Professor of Health Policy and Management, University of Pittsburgh

ANUPAM JENA, Associate Professor of Health Care Policy and Medicine, Harvard Medical School; Assistant Physician, Massachusetts General Hospital

TRACY LIEU, Director, Division of Research, Kaiser Permanente Northern California

GARY LYMAN, Professor of Medicine, University of Washington School of Medicine; Professor, Divisions of Public Health Sciences and Clinical Research, Fred Hutchinson Cancer Research Center

KAVITA PATEL, Fellow, The Brookings Institution

HAROLD PAZ, Executive Vice President and Chancellor for Health Affairs, The Ohio State University, Chief Executive Officer, Ohio State University Wexner Medical Center

DEBORAH SCHRAG, Chief, Division of Population Sciences, Medical Oncology, Dana-Farber Cancer Institute; Professor of Medicine, Harvard Medical School

YA CHEN TINA SHIH, Professor of Health Economics, Department of Health Services Research, The University of Texas MD Anderson Cancer Center

KENNETH SILVERMAN, Director of Packaging Technology, Global Technical Operations, AstraZeneca

HOLLY TAYLOR, Research Bioethicist, Department of Bioethics, Clinical Center, National Institutes of Health

JONATHAN WATANABE, Professor of Clinical Pharmacy and Associate Dean of Assessment and Quality, University of California, Irvine, School of Pharmacy and Pharmaceutical Sciences

ALASTAIR WOOD, Emeritus Professor of Medicine and Pharmacology, Vanderbilt University

K. ROBIN YABROFF, Senior Scientific Director, American Cancer Society

NOTE: See Appendix E, Disclosure of Unavoidable Conflicts of Interest.

Study Staff

FRANCIS KWADWO AMANKWAH, Study Director
ALEXANDRA ANDRADA, Associate Program Officer
ANNALEE GONZALES, Administrative Assistant
TRACY A. LUSTIG, Senior Program Officer
MICAH WINOGRAD, Financial Officer
ANNE MARIE HOUPPERT, Senior Librarian
SHARYL J. NASS, Senior Director, Board on Health Care Services

Consultants

ADITI P. SEN, Johns Hopkins Bloomberg School of Public Health
HUI ZHAO, The University of Texas MD Anderson Cancer Center

Editorial Consultant

ROBERT POOL

Reviewers

This Consensus Study Report was reviewed in draft form by individuals chosen for their diverse perspectives and technical expertise. The purpose of this independent review is to provide candid and critical comments that will assist the National Academies of Sciences, Engineering, and Medicine in making each published report as sound as possible and to ensure that it meets the institutional standards for quality, objectivity, evidence, and responsiveness to the study charge. The review comments and draft manuscript remain confidential to protect the integrity of the deliberative process.

We thank the following individuals for their review of this report:

LINDSEY B. AMERINE, University of North Carolina Eshelman School of Pharmacy
GERARD ANDERSON, Johns Hopkins Center for Hospital Finance and Management
FRANCIS J. CROSSON, Kaiser Permanente Bernard J. Tyson School of Medicine
STACIE B. DUSETZINA, Vanderbilt University Medical Center
RICHARD G. FRANK, Harvard Medical School
MIREILLE JACOBSON, University of Southern California
MICHELLE M. MELLO, Stanford University School of Medicine and Stanford Law School
DAVID H. PETERS, Johns Hopkins Bloomberg School of Public Health
RINO RAPPUOLI, GSK Vaccines

BRUCE J. ROTH, Washington University School of Medicine in St. Louis
LEE SCHWARTZBERG, University of Tennessee Health Science Center
GAIL WILENSKY, Project HOPE

Although the reviewers listed above provided many constructive comments and suggestions, they were not asked to endorse the conclusions or recommendations of this report, nor did they see the final draft before its release. The review of this report was overseen by **ROBERT D. REISCHAUER,** Urban Institute, and **BRADFORD H. GRAY,** Urban Institute. They were responsible for making certain that an independent examination of this report was carried out in accordance with the standards of the National Academies and that all review comments were carefully considered. Responsibility for the final content rests entirely with the authoring committee and the National Academies.

Acknowledgments

The study committee and the Health and Medicine Division (HMD) project staff take this opportunity to recognize and thank the many individuals who shared their time and expertise to support the committee's work and to inform deliberations.

This study was supported by Funding Opportunity Number CMS-2E2-19-001 from the Centers for Medicare & Medicaid Services, U.S. Department of Health and Human Services (HHS). The contents provided do not necessarily represent the official views of HHS or any of its agencies.

The committee benefited greatly from discussions with individuals who made presentations during the committee's open sessions and participated in the discussions: Corinne Axelrod, Peter Bach, Alexander Bastian, Corbin Bennett, Donald M. Berwick, Amitabh Chandra, Jacqueline Corrigan-Curay, Francis Crosson, Gwen Darien, Stacey Dusetzina, Michael Ganio, Peter Gilbar, Sherry Glied, Kedar Gokhale, Daniel Goldstein, Mireille Jacobson, Ronald Khoury, Prabath Malluwa-Wadu, Richard L. Schilsky, Michael Seiden, Brian Serumaga, and Sarah Shirey-Losso. The committee is very grateful to these presenters for volunteering to share their knowledge, data, and expert opinions with the committee and members of the public who attended the committee's open sessions.

Contents

APPENDIXES

Preface

As a physician in training—and later as a practicing clinician—I can remember well some puzzlement when I observed (or personally performed) a treatment that involved breaking the top off a glass vial (or piercing the rubber cap) and extracting a medication from the vial into a syringe. The subsequent infusion into a vein, or injection into a muscle or under the skin, was of course the primary focus of the activity, but the puzzlement arose because often the entire vial was not required for the dose of treatment that the patient was to receive. I would notice the remaining liquid in the bottom of the vial and realize that many questions arose about the process. What should happen with the remaining liquid? Could I save it for another patient? Under what conditions? If not, how should it be safely discarded? Could I have simply administered the entire vial in order to avoid leaving this excess? Did the remaining liquid have value? If so, who was paying for it? (The patient? The treating organization or clinician? The insurer? The pharmaceutical company?) Was the failure to use the entire vial a serious waste of resources?

I recall that we avoided simply dumping the excess liquid down the sink, but the disposal process was often haphazard, and the questions I considered at the time were seldom discussed. The bulk of the medication was generally administered to the patient, and there seemed to be little reason to be overly concerned about the typically small amount of extra liquid that was left behind in the vial. The vial was generally not too expensive, and there was little focus on the issue of waste.

In recent years, however, there has been an explosion in the use of specialty medications that are produced and distributed in vials—typically chemotherapeutic agents or immunologics. Unlike the vials of the past, these individual vials are often extremely expensive, with prices in the thousands of dollars each. Since many of these medications are dosed based on the individual patient's weight or body surface area, it is common for some medication to be left behind after the needed amount, which can vary significantly among patients, is withdrawn from a vial. Yet, concerns about sterility and environmentally correct preservation of the medications prevent the excess from being saved for future use, leading to its being discarded. Given the unit prices of such vials, it is natural to ask how much is being spent unnecessarily on the liquid treatment that is never actually administered to a patient.

Now that specialty drugs make up about 2 percent of total prescription volume but account for one-half of the overall cost of drugs for the U.S. health care system, it is natural for health insurers, including the Centers for Medicare & Medicaid Services (CMS), to ask whether they are spending more than they should on liquid medications that are delivered in glass vials and dosed based on a patient's body size (weight or body surface area). Since some have estimated that the discarded medications may, on a prorated basis, be costing CMS billions of dollars annually, the question has also drawn the attention of the U.S. Congress. Congress accordingly mandated CMS to commission a study by the National Academies of Sciences, Engineering, and Medicine (the National Academies) to address the question of how the nation might best address the perceived failure of the health system to handle effectively and efficiently the weight-based dosing of medications in glass vials. The Committee on Implications of Discarded Weight-Based Drugs was formed in response to this request from CMS.

As we investigated the issues relevant to this topic, the committee members learned quickly that what at first appeared to be a simple question about vials was actually opening up a complex and varied set of related topics. These topics begin with the development of new drugs, carry through clinical trials and the regulatory process, and inevitably involve not only payers for the medications but also the pharmaceutical manufacturers, intermediaries involved with the storage and distribution requirements for the relevant medications, the purchasers and their clinical practices, and ultimately the administration of treatment. Even the concept of "waste" in this context became a matter for debate and clarification, relating to economic concepts of value and how pricing is determined. Also important were patterns of reimbursement, the role of Medicare Part B (rather than Part D) in the coverage for the most expensive specialty medications, and the implications of unused medications from the perspectives of patients—especially if they lacked comprehensive supplemental (MediGap) insurance under Part B.

I should also mention the importance to the committee of an earlier (2018) National Academies report, *Making Medicines Affordable: A National Imperative*. We found the conclusions and recommendations in that report to be both compelling and highly relevant to our own deliberations. Our committee's recommendations can be viewed as building on insightful work that went before, as is emphasized in this report itself.

The committee was challenged by unexpected and complicated issues that arose as the National Academies' typical study processes encountered the 2020 coronavirus disease 2019 (COVID-19) pandemic. Although we were able to meet face to face in January 2020 for our first meeting and had the pleasure of getting to know one another individually at that time, the remaining meetings, workshops, and report deliberations were all held online. We held virtual public hearings via video telecommunication connections on several occasions, receiving briefings that greatly informed the content of the report and our ultimate conclusions and recommendations.

The release of COVID-19 vaccines in December 2020 offered us confirmatory evidence regarding the problem we were studying and, in particular, the advantages of multi-dose vials. Our last committee meeting, included some discussion (and a few moments of levity) as members commented on the sudden public awareness of the advantages of multi-dose vials. A sixth dose of vaccine was discovered in vials that were meant to include only five doses, thereby allowing one more individual to be vaccinated from each vial. Accordingly, there was elation in the public health community and major news coverage of an issue that readers will find addressed within the pages of this report.

Despite the pandemic that forced us into unusual virtual meeting conditions, we had vibrant discussions and built close collaborative relationships, both among the committee members and with the remarkable staff from the National Academies' Health and Medicine Division who guided us through the process. The National Academies deserve recognition and credit for the way in which they responded to the demand for a technological solution to the requirements of our committee as well as many other National Academies activities that have occurred in 2020.

We accordingly begin our thanks with recognition of our study director, Francis Amankwah, whose energy and commitment to the project were evident throughout. He had an excellent grasp of the issues (having worked on the earlier *Making Medicines Affordable* report), organized our efforts with great skill, and demonstrated an ability to capture in writing what committee members discussed or submitted for inclusion. Assisted by Alexandra Andrada (associate program officer) and Annalee Gonzales (administrative assistant), the team mastered the technology and impressed us all with their skill and camaraderie. We note as well the important oversight roles played by Tracy Lustig (senior program officer) and Sharyl Nass (who directs the Board on Health Care Services at the National Academies), both of whom regularly attended our virtual meetings. We benefited greatly from their wisdom and experience.

The committee (see Appendix D) thanks the many individuals who provided briefings on key topics that we needed to understand or who submitted written comments that informed our deliberations (see Appendix C). We found that much of what we needed to study was not previously well documented in writing, so the testimony of these key individuals was valuable and highly appreciated. The detail provided in the report is largely derived from the information provided by these experts and stakeholders.

Some of the information we needed required additional data analysis, and we are grateful for extensive work performed on the committee's behalf by Aditi Sen (Johns Hopkins Bloomberg School of Public Health) and Hui Zhao (The University of Texas MD Anderson Cancer Center). Much of the discussion in Chapter 3 (and in Appendix B) would not have been possible without their rigorous assessment of the relevant Medicare and IBM MarketScan data that were available to us.

As committee chair I want to express also my sincere thanks to the committee members themselves. It was a wonderful group with whom to work, beautifully balanced with regard to expertise and with a uniform commitment to fulfilling the task at hand—even with the complications introduced into the normal study process by the pandemic. Some of the clinicians on the committee had to excuse themselves for periods of times during a call when they had to address the clinical needs of a coronavirus patient, but they returned to re-immerse themselves quickly in the ongoing discussions. I am grateful for having had the opportunity to work with this superb group of scientists and clinicians.

Edward Shortliffe, *Chair*
Committee on Implications of
Discarded Weight-Based Drugs

Summary

Every year, significant amounts of expensive drugs are discarded. This is due in part to the growing number of prescription drugs that are administered in variable doses (rather than fixed or flat doses) based on a patient's weight or body size. Because of safety considerations, the typical approach for manufacturers in the United States is to package these weight-based medications[1] in single-dose vials that are intended for use by a single patient. These vials contain standard amounts of the drug which typically exceed the required dosages for the average patient. Strict regulations and guidance generally discourage or severely restrict the acceptable time frame for sharing medication from single-dose vials among patients. Many of the weight-based drugs in single-dose vials are among the more expensive drugs on the market, and they are paid for by federal health care programs, private health plans, and patients, who have copayment and coinsurance obligations. For Medicare patients, these drugs are covered under Medicare Part B when they are administered by infusion and injection in physician offices or hospital outpatient departments.

Typically, a health care provider will use a patient's weight to calculate the required dose of a drug and extract the appropriate amount

[1] The committee uses the term *weight-based dosing* to refer to drug dosing based on measures of "body size," including dosing based on either weight or body surface area, which is closely correlated with body weight. Although these two approaches can be distinguished and justified clinically, for the purposes of this report they can be considered under the single term *weight-based*.

from a vial (or sometimes two or more vials, depending on how much each vial holds and how much the patient needs). The unused amount will typically be discarded. Since January 2017, the Centers for Medicare & Medicaid Services (CMS) has required health care providers to report, with a particular code called the JW modifier, the portion of drug from a single-dose vial that is discarded and eligible for payment under the "discarded drug policy." Under this CMS policy, health care providers receive payment for the total amount of drug indicated on the vial or package label of a single-dose product, including that which is discarded. However, health care providers' use of the JW modifier is inconsistent, which makes it difficult for health care payers to determine the amount of discarded drug and the associated payments with any accuracy or certainty. Also, when patients are responsible for drug cost-sharing, their share is based on the full content of the single-dose vial even if they received just a portion of it.

Thus, the current situation is one in which significant—but indeterminate—amounts of expensive prescription drugs are discarded each year. In light of this, the U.S. Congress mandated that CMS should enter into an agreement with the National Academies of Sciences, Engineering, and Medicine (the National Academies) to conduct a study on the federal health care costs, safety, and quality concerns associated with discarded drugs that result from the weight-based dosing of medicines contained in single-dose vials. This report is the response to that charge. It examines the current system for the production, administration, and reimbursement of weight-based drugs in single-dose vials with an emphasis on the economic issues related to discarded drugs, it reviews the responses of various stakeholders who have sought to address the issue of discarded drugs, and it offers recommendations on how the system might be improved while also ensuring patient safety. Box S-1 contains the Statement of Task for the study.

In addition to the study's Statement of Task, CMS specifically required the committee to address some key items as they relate to the Statement of Task:

- Provide a comprehensive assessment of federal health care costs, to both the Medicare program and Medicare beneficiaries, due to billing for wasted drugs and biologicals from single-dose vials.
- Using available data sources, quantify the amount of *waste* associated with single-dose injectable drugs and biologics in billing units and/or proportion of available vial sizes and calculate the associated dollar amounts.
- Identify relevant drugs, vial sizes, dosing practices, and delivery practices most associated with *waste*.

BOX S-1
Statement of Task

An ad hoc committee under the auspices of the National Academies of Sciences, Engineering, and Medicine will examine federal health care costs, safety, and quality concerns associated with discarded drugs resulting from weight-based dosing of medicines contained in single-dose vials. Based on that review, the committee will identify relevant drugs and examine

- Current delivery practices, including manufacturing, storage, and transportation guidelines;
- Guidance from relevant federal agencies to biopharmaceutical manufacturers and distributors;
- Federal drug reimbursement and cost-sharing policies;
- Implications of current dosing practice to patients' safety and quality of care; and
- Financial consequences of discarded drugs.

The committee will issue a report with findings and recommendations to consider in order to reduce waste in the biopharmaceutical supply chain.

- Evaluate dosing strategies that may contribute to or mitigate excessive drug *waste* where possible (e.g., dosing based on weight, body surface area, and institutional rounding/dose capping protocols).
- Investigate manufacturer rationale for developing particular vial sizes and safety standards (such as those from the United States Pharmacopeia) influencing requirements for single-dose versus multi-dose vial development and use.

PUTTING THE STUDY IN CONTEXT

To appreciate what is at stake in the area of weight-based drugs in single-dose vials, it is necessary to consider the larger context of health care in the United States. Americans pay significantly more for health care than people in any other country of the world; the percentage of the gross domestic product that the United States devotes to health care is, on average, about twice that of other developed countries even though the health of American citizens is, by most measures, worse than that of citizens of most other developed countries. U.S. health care costs have been rising steadily at well over the rate of inflation for several decades, and they are projected to continue increasing for the foreseeable future.

Prescription drugs account for approximately 17 percent of the overall health care costs in the United States, and drug costs have been increasing faster than overall health care costs for at least the past few decades. A major driver of the ongoing increases in drug costs is spending on specialty drugs[2]—many of which are weight-based drugs in single-dose vials—which account for half of the overall U.S. expenditures on drugs even though they make up only about 2 percent of the total number of prescriptions written each year. In short, the high and increasing costs of weight-based drugs in single-use vials significantly contribute to the high costs of health care in the United States.

At the level of individual patients, high drug costs can lead to substantial financial hardship even for those who have health insurance. Many weight-based, single-dose vial drugs are very expensive—thousands of dollars per treatment is not unusual. Traditional fee-for-service Medicare beneficiaries pay 20 percent of the billed amount for prescription drugs covered under Part B, with no cap on annual total out-of-pocket expenses on drugs. For Medicare beneficiaries, those without supplemental insurance incur substantially higher out-of-pocket costs than their counterparts with supplemental coverage. Even most individuals with health insurance have deductibles, copayments, or coinsurance to pay. This high patient out-of-pocket spending for medical care may be associated with asset depletion and medical debt, distress and worry about household finances, and trade-offs in paying for routine daily needs, including food and housing. Some patients may delay or forgo needed medical care because of expected out-of-pocket costs.

Historically, prescription drugs have been primarily delivered in two forms—as fixed doses or as weight-based doses. In the case of fixed doses, which are typical of the drugs sold in pharmacies, usually in the form of tablets or capsules, patients receive drug doses that may vary by therapeutic need but are not based on a patient's weight. By contrast, weight-based doses, which are typically liquids given through injection or infusion directly by physicians or other health care providers, vary according to a patient's weight or body size and are much more common for infused and injectable drugs than for tablets or capsules. Despite the widespread use of weight-based dosing, particularly in cancer medicine, empirical evidence supporting this practice is limited.

Weight-based dosing has the advantage of being tailored to a patient weight or body size, but this individualization makes manufacturing and

---

[2] *Specialty drugs* is a general term for drugs that feature one or more of the following characteristics: great expense, molecular complexity (often derived from living cells), limited availability or specialized distribution network, unique storage or shipment requirements, and use for treating rare and complex disease indications.

packaging of drugs more complex. Injected or infused drugs are typically packaged in vials intended to be used a single time for a single patient, but because the doses will vary by patient, the drug manufacturer needs to decide which fixed vial size or sizes to produce. No matter what sizes are chosen, some drug will almost always be left over when the appropriate amount is withdrawn from the vial for a treatment. The drugs can be packaged in larger vials intended for multiple uses by multiple patients, but that choice has its own concerns, such as the risk of bacterial contamination after first use and the fact that these drugs can be used only for a limited, specified period of time after the seal has been broken.

In economic terms there is a major difference between fixed-dose and weight-based drugs. That is, with the former, patients receive all of the amount of drug that they pay for and variations in dose are achieved by using multiple pills at a time or an alternate formulation in which there is a higher or lower dose. But for the latter, drug companies generally sell the drug by the vial and even if a patient does not receive the entire contents of a vial, the entire vial still has to be paid for.

This situation, in which the cost of an entire single-dose vial is reimbursed even when only part of the vial is used, provides no incentive to minimize the amount of discarded drug. Because neither drug manufacturers nor health care providers have any incentive to change the system and reduce the amount of discarded drugs, significant amounts of expensive drugs are manufactured and distributed but ultimately not used.

QUESTION OF WASTE

Making appropriate and effective policy choices in this area requires a clear understanding of the concept of drug "waste." The committee's Statement of Task used *waste* specifically to refer to the discarded portions of single-use vials of weight-based drugs, which raised the question of exactly how to understand the term in this context.

While there are many ways to define waste, for the purposes of this report, the most relevant meaning of the term reflects the way it is used by researchers and other observers who are interested in the issue of efficiency in health care spending. In this context, *waste* refers to any spending that does not produce as much value as it could have if it were directed differently, and in this conceptualization of waste, discarded portions of weight-based drugs might fit into the category of clinical waste—assuming that their presence is associated with excessive spending.

On the surface it can indeed seem extremely wasteful that health care providers discard significant portions of the drug in single-dose vials that can cost thousands of dollars. And, indeed, it is that appearance of significant economic waste that has led observers to attempt to calculate the total value of drugs discarded in this way each year and to look for ways to minimize this *waste*. One estimate, for example, indicated that in 2016 approximately $2.8 billion was spent by the federal government and private health care payers on discarded portions of single-use vials of cancer drugs. Another estimate suggested that in 2018, the federal government paid $725 million for discarded drugs administered in hospital outpatient clinics and physician's offices. However, there are a variety of complex factors that could affect the accuracy of how these estimates are made. It is easy enough to multiply the per-milliliter cost of a drug by the number of milliliters discarded each year to get a putative value for how much is "wasted" and then add up all such drugs to get a total, but interpreting that number as the "value" of the discarded drugs is problematic. These typical calculations of the payments for discarded drugs produce only nominal values that are based on the assumption that one can assign a value to an ounce of discarded drug that is equal to the value of an ounce of the drug in an unused vial. They do not accurately capture the "economic value" of discarded drugs and do not reflect the reality of the excess costs to patients and the system. This is because of the factors that go into determining the price of drugs in the United States. The price of a drug is typically based not on how much is used but on the willingness to pay for the drug's therapeutic benefit.

The underlying concern with discarded weight-based drugs is that payers believe that they are paying for discarded medication. One approach to addressing this issue would be to focus on efforts to reallocate unused drugs by sharing vials among multiple patients; another would be to seek reimbursement from manufacturers for these unused drugs. As described in the full report, to the extent that these practices become widespread, drug manufacturers are likely to adjust prices of their drugs upward to reflect the fact that more patients are being treated by the same amount of a given drug, or to account for the cost of reimbursing for unused portions. Raising drug prices combined with the costs associated with developing methods to allocate drugs to multiple patients from single-dose vials or to collect reimbursements would likely not result in any actual financial savings to payers or patients. This would reflect true economic waste in the sense that those resources used to reallocate drugs would not have generated additional medical benefits or cost reductions to payers.

Put differently, because manufacturing costs do not drive drug prices, the quantity of a drug that a patient receives also does not drive pricing. This is why payment strategies used in many other countries provide a uniform reimbursement for a given treatment no matter how much of the drug was required for a specific patient.

Based on the way drugs are priced and paid for in the United States, the committee concluded that when a drug is discarded, there is no money to recoup. Therefore, there is limited economic value to discarded injectable or infused drugs from single-dose vials. While the committee asserts there is little recoverable value to discarded drugs, they do see several opportunities to reduce inefficiencies that could lead to cost savings and improve the quality of care for patients. Therefore, the committee's overarching recommendation[3] is:

> **RECOMMENDATION 5-1: Drug developers, health care providers, and payers should focus their efforts on reducing inefficiencies in drug development, delivery, and payment systems that lead to excess costs for both the health care system and for patients rather than on trying to recoup payments associated with the discarded drugs.**

ALIGNING INCENTIVES AND INCREASING EFFICIENCY TO IMPROVE QUALITY OF CARE

To lay the foundation for strategies to reduce certain inefficiencies that lead to discarded drugs while ensuring patient safety and quality care, the committee presents **two broad goals** and **eight associated recommendations.** The goals and proposed recommendations are oriented toward changing incentives and increasing efficiency in how these drugs are developed, administered, and paid for. The committee recognizes that successfully addressing the issue of discarded drugs will necessitate an implementation process that requires effective collaborations and efforts by all stakeholders in the biopharmaceutical supply chain. Therefore, in formulating its recommendations the committee has considered the ways in which a proposed action could change if another is not carried out. In this sense the committee's recommendations should ideally be viewed as a "package." The two goals are:

- Promote the effective, efficient, and safe use of infused or injectable drugs.
- Implement an efficient and effective reimbursement system for the clinician administration of infused or injected drugs.

---

[3] The committee's recommendations are numbered according to the chapter of the main report in which they first appear. Thus, Recommendation 5-1 is in Chapter 5.

Goal 1: Promote the Effective, Efficient, and Safe Use of Infused or Injectable Drugs

The current practice of using weight-based dosing for many drugs has its roots in historical concerns about balancing the therapeutic actions of a drug against its toxic side effects. When a dosing regimen based on body size (e.g., body surface area or weight) is used in pivotal studies as part of the drug development process, or submitted for registration by an individual or an entity that pays for a clinical trial and collects and analyzes the data, then that regimen will be approved by the U.S. Food and Drug Administration (FDA). Pivotal trials are intended to provide the evidence and data that FDA ultimately uses to decide whether to approve a potential new medicine. Alternatives to weight-based dosing might be just as safe and effective, but weight-based dosing is seldom compared with alternative dosing in pivotal trials. Trials that consider different dosing strategies (e.g., weight-based versus fixed-dose) early in the drug development process could help to determine if dosing based on a patient's body size provides greater benefit than a fixed dose for a given therapeutic agent.

RECOMMENDATION 2-1: The U.S. Food and Drug Administration should require sponsors of pivotal trials for new or extended therapeutic indications to use fixed dosing for a given clinical indication unless safety and efficacy would be compromised. Manufacturers of products already in the market should consider conducting additional studies after approval so that these drugs can, when indicated, be converted to fixed dosing.

Different U.S. agencies have settled on different approaches to single-dose vials. The major reason for not using vials for multiple patients is concerns about compromised sterility and cross-contamination or storage issues once the seal on the container has been broken. Currently, the safety concerns from FDA, CMS, and the Centers for Disease Control and Prevention (CDC), which motivate the regulatory guidance on administering and repackaging of single-dose drugs—that is, dividing the content of a single-dose vial into multiple individual doses—are in conflict. CDC suggests that vials labeled by the manufacturer as single-dose or single-use should only be used for one patient and that repackaging is not acceptable, while FDA and CMS allow for repackaged doses if each one is used only for a single patient. The situation would be greatly improved if the current inconsistent regulatory guidelines were harmonized—and, preferably, modeled on successful protocols in other countries that allow vials to be used for multiple patients.

A number of other Organisation for Economic Co-operation and Development (OECD) countries have well-established clinical and operational approaches that allow for delivering medication to multiple patients from a single vial through vial sharing. Several other countries have promoted standardized doses. For example, dose banding, a system in which drug doses that fall within predefined ranges established through clinical calculations are rounded up or down, is widely used in the United Kingdom and other parts of Europe. Such upward or downward rounding is typically designed to allow use of a complete vial, without discarding any medication.

RECOMMENDATION 2-2: The Secretary of the U.S. Department of Health and Human Services should direct the Centers for Medicare & Medicaid Services, the U.S. Food and Drug Administration, and the Centers for Disease Control and Prevention to work with the United States Pharmacopeia and other nonfederal partners, pharmacists, and infectious disease experts to review and harmonize existing policies and guidelines on drug administration and repackaging. These policies and guidelines should be informed by the successful experiences from other industrialized countries in reducing the amounts of discarded drugs.

RECOMMENDATION 4-1: The Secretary of the U.S. Department of Health and Human Services should direct the Centers for Medicare & Medicaid Services, the U.S. Food and Drug Administration, and the Centers for Disease Control and Prevention to initiate a partnership with other agencies, including the U.S. Department of Defense and the U.S. Department of Veterans Affairs, to work with health care and other organizations with expertise in areas such as industrial design and systems engineering to identify and implement technological systems that allow single-dose vials to be used safely across multiple patients.

RECOMMENDATION 4-2: The Secretary of the U.S. Department of Health and Human Services (HHS) should develop and implement policies that require drug manufacturers to produce injectable and infused drugs in multi-dose vials when it is safe to do so. The Secretary of HHS should routinely review and evaluate the impact of such policies.

Goal 2: Implement an Efficient and Effective Reimbursement System for Clinician Administration of Infused or Injected Drugs

Under the current system for producing, administering, and paying for drugs, health care providers do not have incentives that encourage the efficient use of infused or injectable drugs from single-dose vials. They receive payment for the amount of drug indicated on the label of a single-dose vial, including that which is discarded. This lack of incentives could discourage efforts to reduce the amount of discarded drugs. Also, when patients are responsible for drug cost-sharing, their share is based on the full content of the single-dose vial even if they received just a portion of it.

The committee identified additional problems with the current reimbursement system for clinician administration of infused or injected drugs. For example, Medicare and private payers reimburse health care providers based on the drug's average sales price plus a percentage add-on for administering it. Because the dollar amount of the add-on is larger when the drug price is higher, this system may incentivize clinicians to prescribe more expensive drugs. Addressing these issues will require re-aligning incentives for clinicians' selection and administration of infused or injected drugs.

RECOMMENDATION 2-3: The Secretary of the U.S. Department of Health and Human Services should require the Centers for Medicare & Medicaid Services (CMS) to uncouple add-on payments to clinicians for infused or injected drugs under Medicare Part B from the drug average sales price, focusing the add-on payment instead on CMS's assessment of the time and complexity of drug management and safety monitoring.[4]

RECOMMENDATION 2-4: The Secretary of the U.S. Department of Health and Human Services should require the Center for Medicare & Medicaid Innovation to design and evaluate new payment models that reimburse health care providers by treatment episode rather than by the volume or cost of a drug vial. Findings from the demonstrations should be disseminated widely to other relevant federal agencies, private payers, purchasers, clinicians, and consumers.

In theory, the use of the JW modifier should enable CMS to track the amounts of various drugs discarded from single-dose vials. In practice,

[4] The text in this recommendation was modified since the prepublication release of this report to improve technical accuracy of the language around payments to clinicians for infused or injected drugs under Medicare Part B.

however, a number of limitations exist. The level of compliance with JW coding is highly variable. Not all health care providers use the JW modifier, and among those health care providers that use the modifier, the JW modifier is not reported consistently. Compliance with the JW modifier requirement would enable CMS to track the amount of drug that is discarded from single-dose vials but does not offer practical ways to reduce the amount of discarded drugs. Some observers have argued that enforcing the requirement for using the JW modifier would lead to increased transparency regarding payments for discarded drugs. Others, however, argue that the JW modifier provides an economic incentive for discarding drugs and hinders efficient ways to distribute or administer drugs because it still allows health care providers to be reimbursed regardless of whether all of the drug is actually used. In addition, there are many situations in which drugs are discarded but the JW modifier is not applicable, such as when a drug is administered in a rural health center or a federally qualified health center, because such institutions are generally not separately payable under Part B. In short, the use of the JW modifier appears to be neither consistent nor universal, which makes it impossible to accurately determine the total amounts of discarded drugs or their associated payments each year.

RECOMMENDATION 3-1: While the current Medicare Part B drug reimbursement system is in place, the Centers for Medicare & Medicaid Services should discontinue the use of the JW modifier.

Several versions of draft congressional legislation focused on discarded drugs from single-dose drug vials have proposed rebates from manufacturers to health care providers and payers for discarded drug amounts. However, most bills do not propose refunds directed to patients, who would continue to have cost-sharing responsibilities for portions that were not used in their care. Based on the committee's assessment, it is not feasible to use rebates for discarded drugs to recoup significant funds that could be spent on other health care services, so manufacturer rebates for unused drug are unlikely to achieve the intended aim. Also, given the variety of ways that drugs are priced and reimbursed, a rebate system for clinician-administered drugs would likely be quite complex. Because the committee's assessment shows that there is limited economic value to discarded drugs from single-dose vials under the current system in which drugs are developed, administered, or paid for, a rebate strategy seems unlikely to achieve the intended goals. However, if the rebates that have been proposed in legislation are indeed implemented, the committee asserts that patients need to be included in those rebates.

RECOMMENDATION 4-3: In the event that legislation is enacted or regulatory action is taken to require rebates from manufacturers for discarded drugs, the U.S. Congress should require that rebates be directed first to cover the patient's out-of-pocket expense for the discarded drug and thereafter to health care providers and payers.

INTERDEPENDENCIES OF RECOMMENDATIONS

The nation's biopharmaceutical sector—including the researchers who develop and test drugs, drug manufacturers and distributors, pharmacies, the hospitals and health care providers who administer the drugs, the payers (such as Medicare and private health plans), and the various agencies that regulate drug development, manufacture, use, and reimbursement—is a complex, interconnected system. Changes in one part of the system inevitably affect other parts, often in unanticipated or even undesirable ways. Those looking to implement the recommendations in the report should keep this in mind and be aware of how a proposed change in one area may also affect other areas.

Policy makers should also note that this report's recommendations are interdependent, although their interrelationships vary. In some cases, two or more recommendations are designed to have similar effects, such as the multiple recommendations intended to move the system away from the current standard practice of discarding whatever drug is left in a vial after a single patient has been treated with a portion of the drug rather than sharing the vial among patients. In other cases, recommendations may focus on different issues. The ultimate goal of Recommendation 2-4, for instance, is to create a more equitable payment system. If this goal is met, Recommendation 4-3 may not be necessary. But until that payment system is achieved, the recommendation to cover patients' out-of-pocket expenses with manufacturer rebates is intended to keep the system as fair as possible so that patients are included among those who would benefit from such rebates (see Figure S-1).

Also, consider Recommendations 2-1 and 4-2. Both strive to promote the effective use of infused or injectable drugs in efficient and safe ways but feature different approaches. The ultimate goal of Recommendation 2-1 is to reduce the proportions of the content of vials that are discarded. Fixed doses reduce the proportion of drugs that are discarded but would not completely eliminate leftover drug. For example, in the case where different amounts of fixed doses are used for different indications of a drug that is available only in a vial that is sized for one of those indications, some drug may still be discarded. However, weight-based dosing results in a wide range in doses and amount of drug needed per patient. Consequently, it is almost certain that there will be remaining drug in

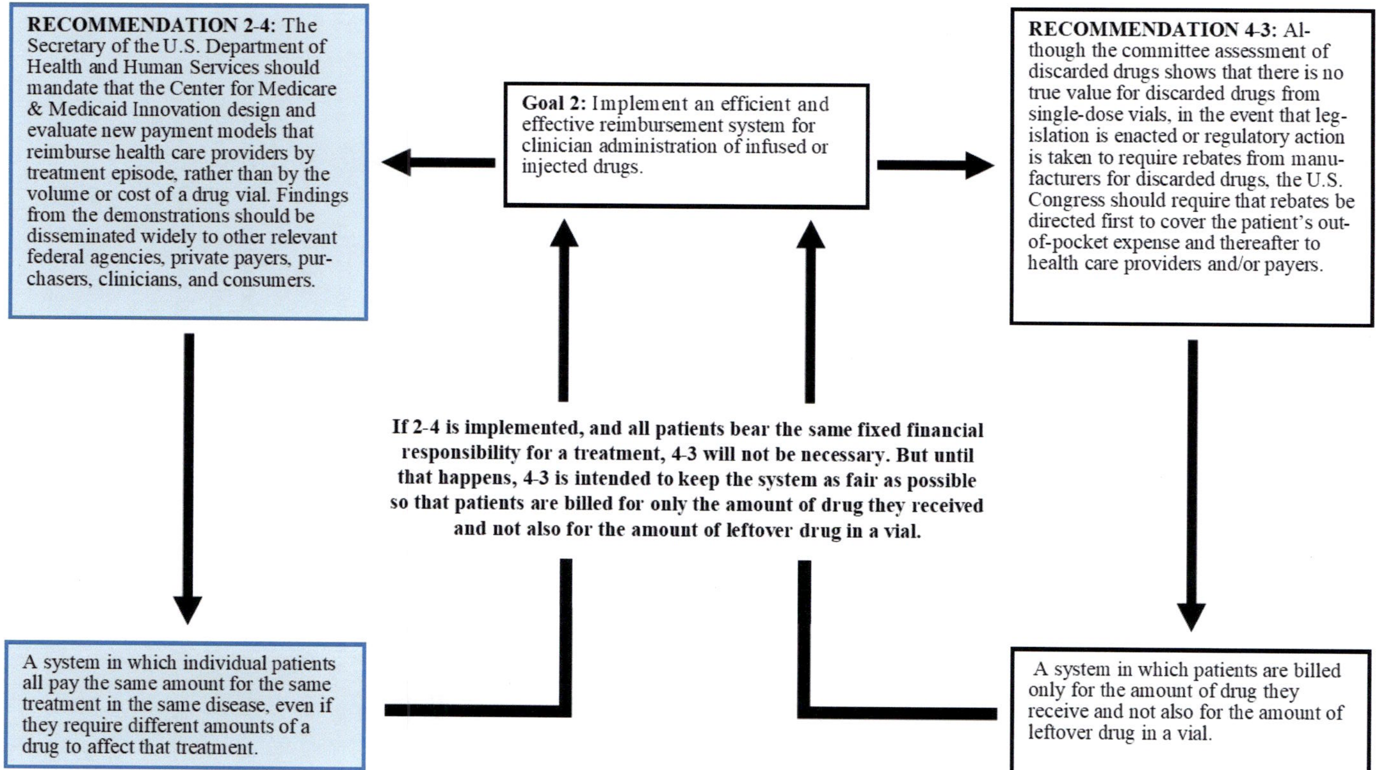

FIGURE S-1 A representation of how two recommendations focus on different issues but are intended to have similar effects by moving the system away from the current standard practice.

the vial. The goal of Recommendation 4-2 is to reduce the proportions of drugs discarded by allowing the content of a vial to be used for more than one patient. If this recommendation is implemented, Recommendation 2-1 may not be necessary.

Policy makers need to be aware of and prepared for the possibility of unintended consequences of implementing new policies. For example, as long as drug manufacturers have near-total freedom to set drug prices, they will likely react to policies that reduce their profits. Thus, if Recommendation 4-3 is adopted, and rebates from manufacturers for discarded drugs are directed to patients to cover their out-of-pocket expense, manufacturers may respond by increasing the price of individual vials so that the profit margins they realize from a particular drug remain approximately the same. Another potential unintended consequence is that the widespread use of multi-dose vials envisioned in Recommendation 4-2 could give an advantage to larger medical centers, where there are more likely to be multiple patients who need the same drug at approximately the same time and thus can jointly receive the contents of a multi-dose vial. Smaller centers would be less likely to benefit due to vials' expiration between recipients.

While the committee's recommendations aim to achieve greater efficiencies in the manufacturing, distribution, and use of injected or infused drugs, it is not possible to predict how much, if any, financial savings might be associated with implementing those recommendations in the absence of additional data for economic analyses. The case for these recommendations is based mainly on nonfinancial considerations, such as safety and equity and overall efficiency.

The Pervasive Issue of Drug Pricing

One of the clearest lessons to be learned from this investigation into weight-based drugs is the burden that these costly drugs places on many patients who rely on these drugs to extend or save their lives. Regardless of whether some portion of a drug vial is discarded, the resulting economic hardship for many Americans due to the prices of these expensive drugs is important. High prescription drug costs are particularly burdensome for older Americans in the Medicare population who often have multiple chronic conditions, such as cancer, rheumatoid arthritis, multiple sclerosis, and other immune disorders, as well as for individuals who are unfortunate enough to develop a disease whose treatment requires more expensive drugs.

Ultimately, ensuring drug affordability will require a much broader and more sustained effort, of the sort described in the 2018 National Academies report *Making Medicines Affordable: A National Imperative*, which put forward a range of proposals to help prevent biopharmaceutical expenditures from spiraling out of control without discouraging continued innovation in drug development. This committee endorses the proposals in that previous National Academies report. In short, the set of recommendations offered in this report would yield significant results if they are leveraged with other strategies aimed at lowering drug prices. Because of various factors such as our aging society and the rising cost of health care, it is more important than ever that the United States act now to address these issues.

1

Introduction

A growing number of prescription drugs, including some of the most expensive ones, are dispensed in variable doses that are administered based on a patient's weight or body surface area (BSA) rather than in fixed or flat doses. Fixed or flat doses of prescription drugs are familiar to patients who have taken antibiotics, pain medications, cholesterol-lowering drugs, and other medications in pill or tablet form; by contrast, many cancer drugs are administered by weight. Such medications have no such thing as a standard dose. Instead, each patient receives a personalized dose based on his or her weight or body size. Because of safety considerations, the typical approach in the United States is to package these medications in single-dose vials that are intended for use by a single patient. This leads to a situation that has been seen by many as a major concern: discarded drugs. Single-dose vials come only in a limited number of specific sizes,[1] so the amount of the drug contained within a vial often exceeds the required weight-based dosage[2] for a given patient, and whatever amount is left over will be discarded. In some cases, that is a significant percentage of the vial. This situation has garnered a great deal of attention because a simple calculation, multiplying the nominal per-milliliter cost of these drugs by the number of milliliters discarded

[1] The phrase *"vial size"* used throughout this report refers to the volume per vial of a drug.

[2] Hereafter, the committee uses *weight-based dosing* to refer to drug dosing based on measures of "body size," including dosing based on either weight or BSA, which is closely correlated with body weight. Although these two approaches can be distinguished and justified clinically, for the purposes of this report, both are considered under the single phrase *"weight-based."*

each year, yields an apparent result of a value in the billions of dollars. The natural question becomes whether it could be possible to save billions of dollars per year by finding a way to avoid discarding these drugs.

STUDY CHARGE

In light of this issue and others related to discarded drugs, the U.S. Congress mandated that the Centers for Medicare & Medicaid Services (CMS) should enter into an agreement with the National Academies of Sciences, Engineering, and Medicine (the National Academies) "to conduct a study on the federal health care costs, safety, and quality concerns associated with discarded drugs that result from weight-based dosing of medicines contained in single-dose vials."[3] The National Academies appointed the Committee on Implications of Discarded Weight-Based Drugs to carry out this task. The full Statement of Task for the committee is presented in Box 1-1.

In addition to the study's formal Statement of Task, CMS required the committee to address some key items as they relate to the Statement of Task.

- Provide a comprehensive assessment of federal health care costs, to both the Medicare program and to Medicare beneficiaries, due to billing for *wasted* drugs and biologicals from single-dose vials.
- Using available data sources, quantify the amount of *waste* associated with single-dose injectable drugs and biologics in billing units and/or proportion of available vial sizes and calculate the associated dollar amounts.
- Identify relevant drugs, vial sizes, dosing practices, and delivery practices most associated with *waste*.
- Evaluate dosing strategies that may contribute to or mitigate excessive drug *waste* where possible (e.g., dosing based on weight, BSA, and institutional rounding/dose capping protocols).
- Investigate manufacturer rationale for developing particular vial sizes and safety standards (such as those from the United States Pharmacopoeia) influencing requirements for single-dose versus multi-dose vial development and use.

Although the committee acknowledges the importance of discarded drugs as it pertains to other drugs—including outpatient prescription

[3] See Committee on Appropriations bill (S. 3040) for the fiscal year ending September 30, 2017. See https://www.congress.gov/114/crpt/srpt274/CRPT-114srpt274.pdf (accessed August 31, 2020).

BOX 1-1
Statement of Task

An ad hoc committee under the auspices of the National Academies of Sciences, Engineering, and Medicine will examine federal health care costs, safety, and quality concerns associated with discarded drugs resulting from weight-based dosing of medicines contained in single-dose vials. Based on that review, the committee will identify relevant drugs and examine

- Current delivery practices, including manufacturing, storage, and transportation guidelines;
- Guidance from relevant federal agencies to biopharmaceutical manufacturers and distributors;
- Federal drug reimbursement and cost-sharing policies;
- Implications of current dosing practice to patients' safety and quality of care; and
- Financial consequences of discarded drugs.

The committee will issue a report with findings and recommendations to consider in order to reduce waste in the biopharmaceutical supply chain.

drugs covered under Medicare Part D that are oral or self-administered—this report focuses on weight-based, single-dose vials covered under Medicare Part B, which are typically administered by clinicians in physician offices and hospitals' outpatient departments by infusion or injection. This report and its conclusions may be relevant to situations in which private health insurance payers use similar methods to reimburse providers for drug administration, but the charge limits the committee's purview to federal programs.

COMMITTEE'S APPROACH

The study committee contained individuals with various areas of expertise, including public health, health care access and affordability, health economics and finance, health care delivery, health care services research, pharmacy, federal health care payment policy, ethics and health care policy, drug manufacturing and packaging, oncology, U.S. Food and Drug Administration (FDA) oversight, and private health insurance. (See Appendix D for the biographical information on the committee and staff.) The committee conducted an extensive review of the literature pertaining to this topic, supplementing it with a variety of sources—including three public information-gathering sessions and written comments from interested stakeholders. The committee also commissioned two analyses: one examining Medicare data intended to help the committee better understand the financial burden of discarded weight-based drugs for the Medicare program and the other examining MarketScan claims linked to Health Risk Assessment data, to help the committee to better understand the financial burden of discarded weight-based drugs for payers and patients in the private health insurance market. The committee also drew on the 2018 National Academies report *Making Medicines Affordable: A National Imperative* (NASEM, 2018).

In this report, the committee uses the phrase *single-dose vials* to refer to drug vials that contain approximately one dose and are intended to be used a single time for a single patient. The committee recognizes that *single-dose vials* and *single-use vials* have been commonly used interchangeably in the literature to mean vials that contain drugs for a single patient. The use of *single-dose vial* is consistent with the approach taken from FDA (2018). The committee uses *multiple-dose vial* to refer to any vial that contains more than one dose of a drug and is intended to be administered multiple times, to either the same or different patients. In 2018, FDA began using a new phrase, *single-patient-use vial*, to describe a vial that contains multiple doses of an injectable medical product and is intended to be used in a single patient (FDA, 2018). The committee chose not to use this label, preferring to employ *multiple-dose vial* for any vial that contains more than one dose of a drug and is intended to be administered multiple times; because the focus of this report is on single-dose vials, the committee saw little utility in introducing an additional term to distinguish between types of multiple-dose vials.

The committee uses *weight-based dosing* to refer to drug dosing based on measures of "body size," including based on either weight or BSA, which is closely correlated with body weight. The committee recognizes that *weight-based dosing* has been used at times in slightly different senses in the literature. Dosage adjustment in children is not addressed in this report, in light of its focus on Medicare Part B. However, the findings and recommendations of this report may well be used by policy makers and the health care industry beyond Medicare Part B.

Additionally, while the main focus of the report is on Medicare Part B, which involves primarily administered and injected drugs, not drugs for which the physician typically writes a "prescription" for a drug to be directly acquired by the patient, this report uses the term *prescription drugs* in a broader sense to indicate all drugs whose use is directed by a physician.

CONTEXT OF RISING HEALTH CARE COSTS

The issue of discarded weight-based drugs from single-dose vials takes place in the larger context of concerns about skyrocketing drug prices and, more generally, about the high cost of health care in the United States. *Making Medicines Affordable* documented that Americans spend, on average, twice as much on health care as people in other high-income countries. Currently, approximately 18 percent of the U.S. gross domestic product (GDP) is spent on health care—a portion that is significantly greater than any other country in the world (NASEM, 2018; Papanicolas et al., 2018).

However, despite this high health care spending, the health of Americans is not noticeably better than that of people living in other wealthy nations, and by many measures it is worse (Papanicolas et al., 2018). For example, according to the World Health Organization's (WHO's) Global Health Observatory data, when countries are ranked by life expectancy, the United States is only 34th on the list, behind several middle-income countries (WHO, 2020). Much of the greater life expectancy in other countries can be attributed to evidence that individuals in other high-income countries tend to have healthier lifestyles than Americans and that these countries generally place greater emphasis on public health practices and social needs—an indication that most other countries are getting a much greater return on their health care spending, in terms of the citizen health, than the United States is (Papanicolas et al., 2018). Furthermore, because the United States is projected to have a steadily aging population over the coming decades, it seems likely that the percentage of GDP spent on health care will continue to increase for the foreseeable future unless some fundamental changes are made in the health care system (NASEM, 2018).

Prescription Drug Expenditures

Many factors contribute to the high costs of U.S. health care, but spending on prescription drugs is a major component of the problem. *Making Medicines Affordable* (NASEM, 2018) described the steady rise in the cost of prescription drugs that has taken place in the United States over the past few decades and discussed the reasons for that rise. As of 2016, prescription drugs accounted for approximately 17 percent of the total cost of U.S. health care services (Kesselheim et al., 2016), and such drugs have been—and continue to be—significant for the increasing health care costs.

In particular, specialty drugs have played a major role in the rapidly rising costs of drugs. Many specialty drugs (which include weight-based injectable and infused drugs) are used for treating different types of cancers and diseases of older persons and are administered in a physician's office or hospital (Lotvin et al., 2014). Currently, while specialty drugs comprise only about 2 percent of the prescriptions written annually in the United States, they account for about one-half of the total U.S. drug spending (IQVIA, 2019).

Given the rapidly rising costs of prescription drugs in the United States, the significant part of overall health care spending that they represent, and the fact that Americans pay so much more for prescription drugs than those in other countries (Kanavos et al., 2013; Sarnak et al., 2017), steps to lower drug costs or slow the increases in those costs could be an important part of the solution to the broader problem of rising health care costs. It was against this backdrop that the committee took on the task of determining whether efforts to reduce "waste" associated with discarded drugs resulting from weight-based dosing of drugs contained in single-dose vials, or to increase efficiency in the dispensing of such drugs, holds promise in that broad effort.

Medicare Part B

The U.S. government has health care programs that serve older persons, persons with disabilities, low-income individuals, veterans, active-duty military personnel and their dependents, and Native Americans. The populations these programs serve, the types of health care services they cover, and, specifically, their prescription drug coverage influence the trends in drug use and spending across these programs. Medicare Part A covers inpatient hospital costs, whereas Part B covers outpatient care and certain drugs—primarily infusible and injectable drugs and biologics—if they are administered in physician's offices and hospital outpatient departments and certain other drugs provided by pharmacies and suppliers. Medicare Part B also covers some outpatient prescription drugs, mainly certain oral cancer and antiemetic drugs that are exact replacements for covered infusible drugs (ASPE, 2020). Medicare Part D covers most outpatient prescription drugs, which patients typically administer themselves.

In Medicare Part B, the health care provider or facility (clinic, physician office, or hospital) buys drugs directly from manufacturers or from intermediaries such as wholesalers or specialty pharmacies, stores them in its practices, and administers them to a patient as needed. The health care provider then submits a claim to either Medicare or the patients' health insurance for reimbursement. The Medicare Modernization Act (MMA) of 2003 changed Medicare's payment methodology for drugs covered by Part B from an average wholesale-price-based approach to a market-based price approach, which is based on the drug's average sales price (ASP) plus a percentage add-on for administering the drug.[4] The ASP is computed using the manufacturer's unit sales of a drug to all U.S. purchasers submitted to CMS in a calendar quarter divided by the number of units sold, minus all price concessions, such as volume discounts, cash discounts, and rebates. Under the budget sequestration cuts, payments to health care providers for most Part B drugs were changed from the ASP plus 6 percent to the ASP plus 4.3 percent (Werble, 2017).

Drug spending has been growing more rapidly in the Medicare Part B program than in any other federal health care program (ASPE, 2020). In 2020, the Medicare Payment Advisory Commission (MedPAC), an independent commission established to advise Congress on issues affecting the Medicare program, released a report that included an analysis of Medicare Part B spending from 2005 to 2018 (MedPAC, 2020). While these data were not adjusted for inflation or the number of enrollees, the analysis found that spending on Medicare Part B drugs increased from $13.4 billion in 2005 to $35 billion in 2018, for an average annual growth rate of 7.7 percent (see Figure 1-1). Physician offices accounted for 57 percent ($19.9 billion) of the total Medicare Part B drug spending in 2018. Hospital outpatient departments accounted for 38 percent ($13.1 billion), and suppliers—including retail pharmacies that supply classes of oral drugs covered under Part B—accounted for 5 percent ($1.9 billion).

A relatively small number of drugs, most of which are specialty drugs, accounts for a substantial share of Part B spending (ASPE, 2020; GAO, 2015). In 2018 the 10 highest-cost drugs, which mainly treat cancer, macular degeneration, and immune-mediated diseases such as rheumatoid arthritis, accounted for $12.2 billion in Part B payments (not including beneficiary cost-sharing), or 46 percent of the $26.6 billion in total Part B spending for all drugs (ASPE, 2020).

Traditional fee-for-service Medicare beneficiaries pay 20 percent of the Medicare-approved amount for covered Part B prescription drugs (CMS, 2020). Approximately 81 percent of these beneficiaries have supplemental health insurance or drug coverage that is purchased separately, comes from Medicaid, or comes from prior employers (Cubanski et al., 2019). The remaining 19 percent who have no supplemental coverage pay 20 percent coinsurance for Part B drugs, with no cap on annual total-out-of-pocket expenses. The committee recognizes that not all Medicare beneficiaries will use Part B drugs, and most of them have supplemental coverage. However, the way Part B drugs are acquired and paid for places a significant out-of-pocket burden on those who do need Part B drugs

[4] See https://www.congress.gov/bill/108th-congress/house-bill/1 (accessed September 23, 2020).

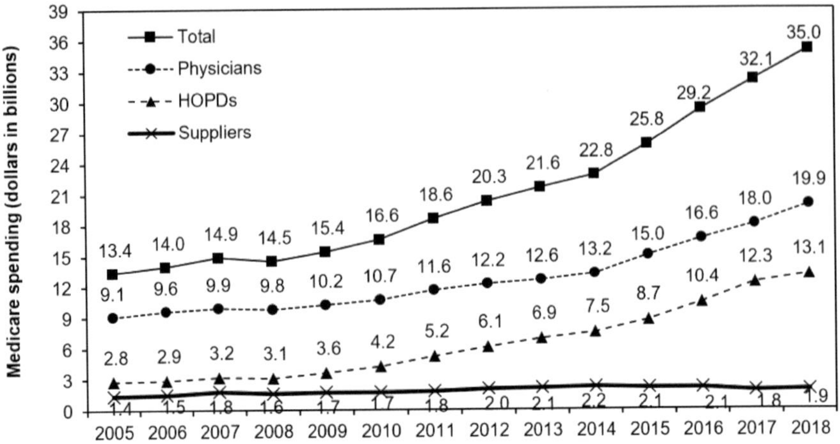

FIGURE 1-1 Medicare spending for Part B drugs furnished by physicians, hospital outpatient departments (HOPDs), and suppliers, 2005–2018.
NOTES: Data include Part B–covered drugs furnished by several provider types including physicians, suppliers, and hospital outpatient departments, and exclude those furnished by critical access hospitals, Maryland hospitals, and dialysis facilities. "Medicare spending" includes program payments and beneficiary cost-sharing. Data reflect all Part B drugs whether they were paid for based on the ASP plus 6 percent or another payment formula. Data exclude blood and blood products (other than clotting factor). Components may not sum to the total due to rounding.
SOURCE: MedPAC, 2020.

and lack supplemental coverage. These individuals are typically older Americans and often on fixed incomes (Jacobson et al., 2017). High patient out-of-pocket spending is associated with financial hardship, asset depletion and medical debt, distress and worry about household finances, and trade-offs in paying for routine daily needs, including food and housing (Ubel et al., 2013; Yabroff et al., 2018; Zheng et al., 2019). Patients may delay or forgo needed medical care because of expected out-of-pocket costs (Briesacher et al., 2007; Laba et al., 2020; Reynolds et al., 2020). Again, while the number of patients affected by high out-of-pocket expenses for Part B drugs may be small, this population may be among the most vulnerable, and the financial burden on those patients to get the care they need may be overwhelming.

Although clinician-administered drugs currently account for a relatively small share of overall spending on prescription drugs, the spending is projected to increase in the coming years because of the rapidly increasing number of specialty medications coming to the market as single-dose vials. The fundamental issues addressed by this report can inform an overarching approach to reducing certain inefficiencies in the system in which drugs are developed, administered, or paid for that lead to discarded drugs and the associated costs and could set a precedent that the rest of the health care sector could adopt.

QUESTION OF WASTE

According to its Statement of Task, the committee was charged to offer findings and recommendations on how to reduce *waste* in the biopharmaceutical supply chain, and given that the committee's work was to focus specifically on the discarded portions of single-dose vials of weight-based drugs, it understood *waste* to be referring specifically to these discarded portions, which raised the question of how to understand the term. WHO uses the phrase *waste pharmaceuticals* to describe drugs that need to be disposed of for various reasons—because they are past their expiration date, for instance, or labeled in a way that makes them unrecognizable (WHO, 1999)—and the discarded portions of weight-based drugs could certainly be described as waste in this sense.

However, the term is used in a different way by researchers and other observers who are interested in the issue of efficiency in health care spending (Bentley et al., 2008; Berwick, 2019). In this context *waste* refers to any spending that does not produce as much value as it could have if it were directed differently. The existence of this sort of waste does not require a physical manifestation (e.g., discarded drugs), as the focus is on inefficiencies of any sort, but discarded drugs or other medical supplies could be an indication of waste. This waste can appear in a variety of forms: administrative waste (e.g., excess overhead costs), operational waste (e.g., duplication of services), and clinical waste (e.g., practices that do not improve health outcomes or are detrimental to the patient) (Bentley et al., 2008). In this conceptualization of waste, discarded portions of weight-based drugs might fit into the category of clinical waste—assuming that these indicated excessive spending.

On the surface, it can seem extremely wasteful that health care providers discard significant portions of a drug in single-dose vials that can cost thousands of dollars. And, indeed, it is that appearance of significant economic waste that has led observers to attempt to calculate the total value of drugs discarded in this way each year and to look for ways to minimize this *waste*. On the other hand, as the committee discovered in its deliberations and discussions with invited speakers to the committee's public session, many economists who examine this system contend that the concept of *waste* is not the appropriate construct for assessing and addressing the issue of discarded drugs. Some even suggest that this seemingly wasteful system of distributing weight-based drugs might actually be reasonably efficient. The reasons, as discussed in greater detail later in the report, can be found in the marginal costs of producing more drugs and in the factors that go into determining their pricing and paying for them.

This state of affairs presented the committee with a conundrum. But what if it is not appropriate to consider the discarded portions of single-dose vials to actually be fiscal waste? The committee's solution was to approach this report as follows. In the next three chapters, the committee examines the issues surrounding discarded portions of weight-based drugs in single-dose vials from various perspectives—manufacturing, clinical, regulatory, and so on—and offers conclusions about some of the weaknesses of the system in which drugs are developed, administered, or paid for. In Chapter 5, the committee examines the economics of these weight-based drugs and, particularly, the issue of whether it is appropriate to consider discarded portions of single-use vials to be waste. Because the Statement of Task specifically charged the committee to look at financial implications, the committee focused on the economic value of discarded drugs. While a fuller discussion appears in Chapter 5, the committee ultimately decided that it is not appropriate to refer to the discarded portions as "waste" and that even if some inefficiency exists in the way these drugs are administered, the total economic value of discarded drug is nowhere near the amounts that have been suggested by simple calculations that multiply the nominal per-milliliter cost of the drugs by the total milliliters discarded each year. Nonetheless, there are important improvements that can be made to the system in which drugs are developed, administered, or paid for, and the committee does offer recommendations for such improvements in subsequent chapters.

STRUCTURE OF THE REPORT

Chapter 2 examines the factors in the U.S. biopharmaceutical supply chain that interact or compete to influence the amount of discarded drugs from weight-based dosing of drugs in single-dose vials and the patient safety and quality-of-care issues related to weight-based drugs. Chapter 3 gives an overview of the amounts of drugs being discarded. Chapter 4 discusses the actions of various stakeholders, including Congress, nongovernmental and professional organizations, and hospitals and clinicians, to reduced discarded drugs resulting from the use of weight-based drugs in single-use vials. As noted earlier, Chapter 5 focuses on the economic issues related to single-dose, weight-based drugs and explains why waste is not the right construct to analyze the issue of discarded drugs. Chapter 6 contains the committee's goals and reiterates its recommendations.

The report's appendixes present supplemental information on conducting the study. Appendix A contains the glossary of key terms used in the report; Box 1-2 provides some of these. Appendix B contains supplemental information for the committee's commissioned analyses. Appendix C lists experts who spoke at the committee's public sessions and organizations that submitted comments on the study. Appendix D provides committee and staff biographies. Finally, Appendix E provides information on the disclosure of unavoidable conflicts of interest.

BOX 1-2
Key Definitions

Average sales price: Derived from the manufacturer's unit sales of a drug to all U.S. purchasers in a calendar quarter divided by the number of units sold, after all discounts and rebates (except Medicaid rebates).

Clinician-administered drug: An outpatient drug other than a vaccine that is typically administered by infusion or injection by a health care provider in a physician's office or other outpatient clinical setting.

Fixed dosing (also known as flat dosing): Refers to dosing strategies that do not take into account body size or other patient-specific pharmacological parameters.

Multiple-dose vial: Intended to contain more than one dose of a drug and to be used multiple times and for multiple patients.

Single-dose vial: Contains one dose of a drug and is intended to be used a single time for a single patient.

Specialty drugs: This is a general term for drugs that feature one or more of the following characteristics: great expense, molecular complexity (often derived from living cells), limited availability or specialized distribution network, unique storage or shipment requirements, and use for treating rare and complex disease indications.

Weight-based dosing: *Weight-based* refers to the dosing strategy that adjusts dose for body weight. For the purposes of this report the committee uses *weight-based dosing* to refer to drug dosing based on measures of "body size," including based on body surface area, which is closely correlated with body weight.

REFERENCES

ASPE (Office of the Assistant Secretary for Planning and Evaluation). 2020. *Report to Congress: Prescription drug pricing*. May 2020. https://aspe.hhs.gov/system/files/aspe-files/263451/2020-drug-pricing-report-congress-final.pdf (accessed October 27, 2020).

Bentley, T. G., R. M. Effros, K. Palar, and E. B. Keeler. 2008. Waste in the US health care system: A conceptual framework. *The Milbank Quarterly* 86(4):629–659.

Berwick, D. M. 2019. Elusive waste: The Fermi paradox in US health care. *JAMA* 322(15):1458–1459.

Briesacher, B. A., J. H. Gurwitz, and S. B. Soumerai. 2007. Patients at-risk for cost-related medication nonadherence: A review of the literature. *Journal of General Internal Medicine* 22(6):864–871.

CMS (Centers for Medicare & Medicaid Services). 2020. *Medicare Part B: Drug average sales price*. https://www.cms.gov/Medicare/Medicare-Fee-for-Service-Part-B-Drugs/McrPartBDrugAvgSalesPrice (accessed August 4, 2020).

Cubanski, J., T. Neuman, S. True, and M. Freed. 2019. *What's the latest on Medicare drug price negotiations?* http://files.kff.org/attachment/Issue-Brief-Whats-the-Latest-on-Medicare-Drug-Price-Negotiations (accessed August 31, 2020).

FDA (U.S. Food and Drug Administration). 2018. *Selection of the appropriate package type terms and recommendations for labeling injectable medical products packaged in multiple-dose, single-dose, and single-patient-use containers for human use guidance for industry*. https://www.fda.gov/media/117883/download (accessed August 8, 2020).

GAO (U.S. Government Accountability Office). 2015. *Medicare Part B: Expenditures for new drugs concentrated among a few drugs, and most were costly for beneficiaries*. GAO-16-12 October. Washington, DC: GAO.

IQVIA Institute for Human Data Science. 2019. *Medicine use and spending in the U.S.: A review of 2018 and outlook to 2023*. https://www.iqvia.com/-/media/iqvia/pdfs/institute-reports/medicine-use-and-spending-in-the-us---a-review-of-2018-outlook-to-2023.pdf?_=1596563978024 (accessed August 8, 2020).

Jacobson, G., S. Griffin, T. Neuman, and K. Smith. 2017. *Income and assets of Medicare beneficiaries, 2016–2035*. https://www.kff.org/medicare/issue-brief/income-and-assets-of-medicare-beneficiaries-2016-2035 (accessed December 16, 2020).

Kanavos, P., A. Ferrario, S. Vandoros, and G. F. Anderson. 2013. Higher U.S. branded drug prices and spending compared to other countries may stem partly from quick uptake of new drugs. *Health Affairs* 32(4):753–761.

Kesselheim, A. S., J. Avorn, and A. Sarpatwari. 2016. The high cost of prescription drugs in the United States: Origins and prospects for reform. *JAMA* 316(8):858–871.

Laba, T. L., L. Cheng, A. Kolhatkar, and M. R. Law. 2020. Cost-related nonadherence to medicines in people with multiple chronic conditions. *Research in Social and Administrative Pharmacy* 16(3):415–421.

Lotvin, A. M., W. H. Shrank, S. C. Singh, B. P. Falit, and T. A. Brennan. 2014. Specialty medications: Traditional and novel tools can address rising spending on these costly drugs. *Health Affairs* 33(10):1736–1744.

MedPAC (Medicare Payment Advisory Commission). 2020. *A data book: Health care spending and the Medicare program*. http://medpac.gov/docs/default-source/data-book/july2020_databook_entirereport_sec.pdf?sfvrsn=0 (accessed August 4, 2020).

NASEM (National Academies of Sciences, Engineering, and Medicine). 2018. *Making medicines affordable: A national imperative*. Washington, DC: The National Academies Press.

Papanicolas, I., L. R. Woskie, and A. K. Jha. 2018. Health care spending in the United States and other high-income countries. *JAMA* 319(10):1024–1039.

Reynolds, E. L., J. F. Burke, M. Banerjee, K. A. Kerber, L. E. Skolarus, B. Magliocco, G. J. Esper, and B. C. Callaghan, 2020. Association of out-of-pocket costs on adherence to common neurologic medications. *Neurology* 94(13):e1415–e1426.

Sarnak, D. O., D. Squires, G. Kuzmak, and S. Bishop. 2017. Paying for prescription drugs around the world: Why is the U.S. an outlier? *Commonwealth Fund Issue Brief* 1–14.

Ubel, P. A., A. P. Abernethy, and S. Y. Zafar. 2013. Full disclosure—out-of-pocket costs as side effects. *New England Journal of Medicine* 369(16):1484–1486.

Werble, C. 2017. *Medicare Part B.* Health Affairs Health Policy Brief. https://www.healthaffairs.org/do/10.1377/hpb20171008.000171/full (accessed November 20, 2020).

WHO (World Health Organization). 1999. *Guidelines for safe disposal of unwanted pharmaceuticals in and after emergencies.* https://www.who.int/water_sanitation_health/medicalwaste/unwantpharm.pdf (accessed November 20, 2020).

WHO. 2020. *The Global Health Observatory. Life expectancy at birth (years).* https://www.who.int/data/gho/data/indicators/indicator-details/GHO/life-expectancy-at-birth-(years) (accessed November 20, 2020).

Yabroff, K. R., J. Zhao, Z. Zheng, A. Rai, and X. Han. 2018. Medical financial hardship among cancer survivors in the United States: What do we know? What do we need to know? *Cancer Epidemiology and Prevention Biomarkers* 27(12):1389–1397.

Zheng, Z., A. Jemal, X. Han, G. P. Guy, Jr., C. Li, A. J. Davidoff, M. P. Banegas, D. U. Ekwueme, and K. R. Yabroff. 2019. Medical financial hardship among cancer survivors in the United States. *Cancer* 125(10):1737–1747.

2

Single-Dose Vials of Weight-Based Drugs

For most injectable or infusible medications, a measured amount of the drug is drawn from a container[1] using calibrated syringes and then given to the patient. Some of these drugs are injected or infused in fixed amounts, with every patient receiving the same dose. However, the dosage of many injectable or infusible drugs, particularly cancer drugs, depends on a patient's weight.[2] In the United States, weight-based drugs are typically supplied in single-dose vials—that is, in vials that are intended to be used by a single patient because of various health-related concerns that arise if multiple patients share a vial. The vials may come in one or several sizes,[3] and depending on size, a single patient may be treated with one or several vials in order to receive the correct dose.

[1] The container could be a glass or plastic bottle often used to store medication as liquids, powders, or capsules. Some containers could contain medication for injection or infusion for a single patient as a single administration at a single time. The remainder is disposed of after use because the vials do not contain preservatives to stop microbial growth. Such types are referred to as *single-dose* or *single-use* containers. They are usually supplied in ampules, small vials, and prefilled syringes. Vials have rubber stoppers that must be pierced with a needle, and their contents can be stored for a relatively short time once opened. Ampules do not have rubber stoppers and the glass neck must be broken; they must not be stored or reused after that. Other types of containers hold medications intended for multiple doses for injection or infusion and for more than one patient. They contain preservatives to stop bacterial growth but can still be contaminated if safe injection practices are not followed. They are usually referred to as *multi-dose vials*.

[2] As noted in Chapter 1, for the purposes of this report, *weight-based dosing* includes dosing based on body surface area.

[3] The phrase *vial size* used throughout this report refers to the volume per vial of a drug.

Generally, a certain amount of drug will be left over because the dose that the patient requires is not exactly equal to the amount of drug contained in one or multiple vials. Typically, the unused drug is discarded—thus, the "discarded drugs" specified in the committee's Statement of Task. This chapter offers an overview of the factors in the U.S. biopharmaceutical supply chain that interact or compete to influence the amount of discarded drugs from weight-based dosing of medicines contained in single-dose vials including the drug discovery and development process, drug dosing approaches, vial sizes, guidance from federal and nongovernmental organizations, and clinician acquisition of and payment for drugs. The chapter concludes with an examination of patient safety and quality-of-care issues related to weight-based drugs.

DRUG DISCOVERY AND DEVELOPMENT PROCESS

Injectable and infusible drugs are delivered in weight-based doses for a variety of reasons, but among the most important is the establishment of this regimen during the drug development process.

The typical time line from drug discovery to development in the United States can be as long as 15 years, and it involves a series of stages, including discovery, preclinical trials, clinical trials, U.S. Food and Drug Administration (FDA) approval, and post-marketing surveillance (see Figure 2-1).

At the beginning of the discovery stage, researchers in academia, government agencies such as the National Institutes of Health, and the biopharmaceutical industry work to understand the underlying causes and potential treatments of a disease. They often test compounds in the laboratory and in animal models to determine which ones show some activity against the targeted disease and are safe enough for human testing. The analyses of the data from this testing must provide detailed information on dosing and toxicity levels. After animal testing and the accompanying analyses, if the drug manufacturer wishes to continue on to perform tests in humans, it must submit an investigational new drug (IND) application to FDA (2015a).[4]

Approval of the IND advances the potential drug to the clinical stage (known as *clinical trials*), where it is presumed safe to be tested in humans. The potential drug is tested in a clinical setting during three phases of trials, usually lasting 6 to 7 years. In Phase I trials, investigators gather information on safety, tolerability, drug metabolism and excretion, side effects, and mechanisms for determining the maximum tolerated dose.

[4] FDA does not develop drugs. Instead, it develops regulations for good laboratory practices and oversees each study to help ensure drug safety.

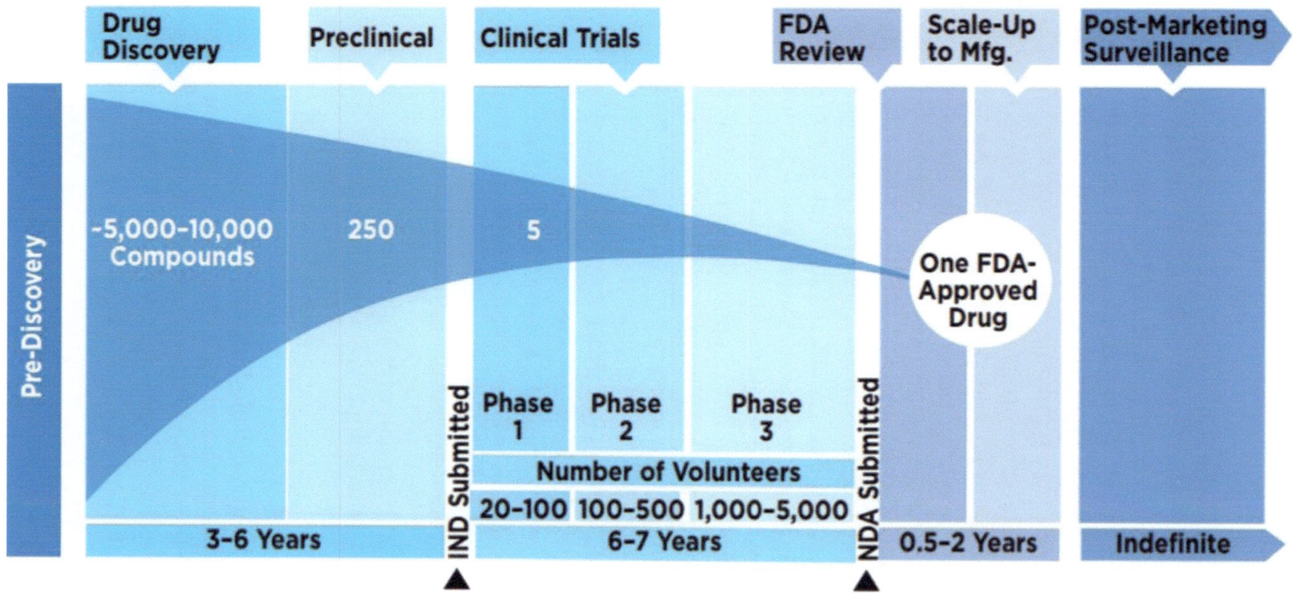

FIGURE 2-1 A typical time line for drug discovery and development in the United States.
SOURCE: NASEM, 2018.

The drug formulation and method of administration may be refined continuously until, and even after, the drug's final approval (FDA, 2018d).

In Phase II trials, investigators gather preliminary information about the potential drug's long-term safety, determine if it has the intended effect in humans, and identify any side effects and any benefits beyond its intended effect (FDA, 2018d). Phase III trials represent the final step in determining if a potential drug is safe and effective (FDA, 2018d). The dosing regimen shown to be safe and effective in these pivotal studies[5] will be the regimen that regulators approve for marketing. The drug manufacturer submits a new drug application to FDA to formally request approval for the drug to be sold and marketed in the United States and for doctors to prescribe it for patients. Typically, for the new drug to be sold in other countries, it would have to satisfy the regulatory requirements in those countries. After the drug is available on the market, further trials—referred to as *Phase IV trials*—may be carried out by the drug's manufacturer; in some cases, FDA requires the manufacturer to carry out further evaluations of the drug's safety or efficacy in order to obtain marketing approval, while in others the manufacturer chooses to carry out the studies to get more information about the drug such as looking for additional indications. Whether or not Phase IV trials are carried out, all drugs are monitored to identify new or delayed toxicity—a process described as *post-marketing surveillance*.

Drug manufacturers may further study the drug in different doses and specific populations, such as older adults or children, and may conduct more research to obtain FDA approval to use it in a new formulation or for another indication, such as another type of cancer. FDA does not make decisions on reimbursement or on how much a drug should cost.

Establishment of Weight-Based Dosing in the Drug Development Process

As noted above, drug doses are established during early clinical trials to demonstrate that the drug is both safe and effective (FDA, 2005; Musuamba et al., 2017). Developing novel therapies often involves early dose-ranging studies in clinical trials that first increase the dose (corrected for body weight) until dose-limiting toxicity occurs and then reduce the dose below that level for pivotal efficacy trials. The dosing regimen tested in these pivotal studies will be the regimen that is approved by FDA.

[5] A pivotal trial or pivotal study is a clinical trial or study that intends to provide the ultimate evidence and data that FDA uses to decide whether to approve a potential new medicine. A pivotal trial is usually a Phase III clinical trial, but in exceptional cases, a Phase II study can serve. They are sometimes also referred to as registration trials.

That is, if a weight-based dosing regimen is used in these pivotal studies, then a weight-based dosing regimen will be approved. Seldom, if ever, do pivotal studies compare a weight-based dosing regimen and a fixed dose. Therefore, an adult dose for many injectable or infusible drugs is frequently weight based because of the early drug development process.

DRUG DOSING

The dosing regimen for a given drug can contribute to the discarding of drugs. One of the main difficulties facing physicians who are attempting to determine the most effective dose of a drug is that different individuals have highly variable abilities to metabolize and eliminate drugs, which means that individuals given comparable doses do not always receive comparable exposures. The use of height and, particularly, weight in determining dose is based on limited preclinical and clinical evidence combined with the general understanding that larger patients have a larger volume of distribution, leading to the presumption that they require a higher dosage to provide the same therapeutic effect. It has been observed, however, that even if doses are adjusted based on body weight, individuals differ in their capacity to metabolize and eliminate drugs due to a combination of physiologic variables, genetic characteristics, and environmental factors, such as food intake and drug–drug interactions (Ahmed et al., 2016; Belle and Singh, 2008; Brunton et al., 2017).

Such variation has received particular attention for anticancer drugs, which often have a steep dose–response relationship and narrow therapeutic index, potentially leading to severe dosing errors (Pai, 2012). To optimize the therapeutic effect, anticancer dosing has historically been guided in both preclinical and early clinical studies by the determination of the "maximum tolerated dose"—that is, the largest dose that a patient can be given before the onset of severe, life-threatening toxicity (Musuamba et al., 2017). This approach for traditional cytotoxic agents has been supported in both preclinical and clinical studies, which have demonstrated that the greater the dose intensity (dose per unit time), the greater the response.

In light of this, new approaches are being explored to determine the optimal therapeutic dose, including dosing based on therapeutic drug monitoring and genotyping of drug-metabolizing capacity or on the area under the plasma concentration curve. The goal is to ensure that sufficiently high local drug concentrations are achieved to maximize efficacy without unacceptable toxicity.

Weight-Based Dosing

Most injectable or infused drugs, especially chemotherapy agents, are dosed according to a patient's body size (e.g., weight, body surface area) because of perceived contribution of body size to individual variations in how drugs are absorbed, distributed, metabolized, and the excreted pharmacokinetic variability (Kaestner and Sewell, 2007; Pan et al., 2016). This practice, however, is uncommon for other medications with sufficiently high therapeutic index, such as antibiotics and allergy medications, for which the dose required for a patient to receive a therapeutic benefit is much lower than the dose necessary to reach the toxic threshold (Tamargo et al., 2015). Based on a 2012 systematic review of FDA-approved drugs, out of 240 systemic drugs, 175 had a weight-based dosing recommendation for adults (Pai, 2012). For some medications, such as hydrocortisone, vancomycin, linezolid, and aprotinin, weight-based dosing has been shown to be superior to other methods for adult patients (Pan et al., 2016). However, weight-based dosing has important limitations for certain populations. For example, because of the lack of specific guidance on limiting toxicity, clinicians may struggle to accurately administer medications to patients with extreme body sizes (Pan et al., 2016). Despite these limitations, the Joint Commission International Accreditation Standards for Hospitals requires that the hospital policy should require weight-based dosing in particular circumstances, such as in pediatric or older patients (Pan et al., 2016).[6]

Among the various dosing strategies that take weight and body composition into account, weight-based dosing is the least consistent across an entire population in terms of the effective dose that individuals receive. Determining a dose solely on the basis of body weight makes an implicit assumption that all individuals have approximately the same body composition, but that is not the case. To address such issues, early-phase clinical trials need, to the extent possible, to include bodies at the extremes of the weight continuum in order to provide the necessary data for determining the appropriate modifications to the strictly body-weight dosing or to dosing determined according to body surface area (BSA), which is a variant of weight-based dosing.

Improving the safety and efficacy of weight-based dosing will require hospitals and other relevant organizations to implement standard operating procedures for weighing patients and creating proper weight documentation, verifying pharmacies' quality control for these dosing regimens, and ensuring the availability of appropriate resources and

[6] It should be noted that body weight increases faster with age in pediatrics, so other dosing methods may be more cost efficient if dosage is based on weight.

functional equipment for necessary health care delivery (Pan et al., 2016). In one study, 46 percent of inpatients receiving a narrow therapeutic index antibiotic did not have their weight documented because of workflow interruptions and heavy workloads (Charani et al., 2015). In another example, a study analyzing administration errors made by physicians and nurses attempting to manually calculate weight-based dosing for an *N*-acetylcysteine regimen for acetaminophen overdose found that 26 percent of the observed calculations were wrong and led to dosing errors (Selvan et al., 2007). By contrast, there was 100 percent accuracy in dose calculations and an improvement in patient safety for those who used an approved weight-based dosing chart. Without proper procedures, inaccurate weight estimates and omitted weight documentation can contribute to dosing errors. A variant of weight-based dosing that takes a patient's body composition into account is BSA-based dosing.

Fixed or Flat Dosing

Fixed dosing (also known as flat dosing) refers to strategies that include no correction for body weight or other pharmacological parameters (Mathijssen et al., 2007). Fixed dosing has long been common in non-oncological treatments, but it has only recently gained increasing use in the oncology field (Hendrikx et al., 2017).

Fixed-dose prescribing has been used for newer targeted therapies covered under Medicare Part B that are highly selective for specific cellular pathways and molecular targets, that demonstrate different relationships between exposure and effect on the molecular target, and that display quite different dose-limiting toxicities than cytotoxic chemotherapy.[7] Fixed dosing of these targeted agents has become standard despite wide inter-individual variation in plasma concentrations following standard dose regimens and substantial interindividual variability in plasma concentration throughout the dosing interval. Such heterogeneity is thought to be due to the genetic heterogeneity of drug targets associated with tumor response and pharmacokinetics factors, including metabolism and oral absorption (bioavailability), environmental factors, and adherence to the regimen. Although oral dosing offers the convenience of self-administration, food intake and drug–drug interactions and adherence have been shown to be challenging, potentially compromising clinical outcomes.

Fixed-dosing approaches offer several advantages over weight-based dosing (Pan et al., 2016), such as greater convenience and safety, with fewer calculations, preparation, and administration errors (Mathijssen et

[7] See https://www.uptodate.com/contents/dosing-of-anticancer-agents-in-adults (accessed September 23, 2020).

al., 2007). Additionally, the ability to use a single vial per patient without the need to discard unused drug could also have a very favorable effect on the expenses associated with anticancer chemotherapy (Hall et al., 2020; Markman, 2005). Fixed dosing lowers stocking and distribution costs and associated complexities. Enhanced patient safety often accompanies fixed-dosing approaches as well.

Like dosing based on body size, fixed chemotherapy dosing is based on clinical trial data from an "average-sized patient." This appears to result in a toxicity profile that is similar to the one obtained with dosing based on weight or BSA for selected cytotoxic agents (Markman, 2005). The optimal dosing of novel selective targeted therapies and immunotherapies remains unclear in many settings. Increasingly, fixed dosing is proving valuable for targeted agents (such as the tyrosine kinase and BRAF inhibitors) and some monoclonal antibodies[8] that target the immune system. For example, in 2014, FDA approved pembrolizumab, a drug used to treat several forms of advanced cancers, to be dosed based on weight (FDA, 2014). Almost 2 years later, new approvals for pembrolizumab to treat different forms of cancer moved from weight-based to fixed dose. Currently, pembrolizumab is given with fixed dosing for all indications (FDA, 2020).

In brief, because of convenience, safety, and the potential cost savings in the manufacture, packaging, and storing of fixed doses, fixed dosing for all patients regardless of body size characteristics has become the standard for essentially all oral targeted therapies.

Other Dosing Practices

Variation in body size characteristics does not adequately explain most interindividual pharmacokinetic variability for anticancer agents, so researchers and clinicians have tried various other dosing practices in an effort to give patients the most effective doses for their individual situations (Brunton et al., 2017). Pharmacokinetics attempts to understand how the body handles drugs, including absorption (for oral drugs), distribution (to different organs/body compartment), metabolism (activation/inactivation by enzymes), and elimination (generally renal or hepatic) (Brunton et al., 2017). Because of interest in more personalized or precision dosing, pharmacogenetic- and pharmacokinetic-based dosing strategies have received considerable attention, although their use in clinical practice has remained limited up to this point.

[8] Monoclonal antibodies are laboratory-produced molecules engineered to serve as substitute antibodies that can restore, enhance, or mimic the immune system's attack on cancer cells. They are designed to bind to antigens that are generally more on the surface of cancer cells than healthy cells.

Therapeutic drug monitoring involves measuring plasma drug concentrations to adjust dosages to achieve optimal drug concentrations. Although it is accepted as a way to guide dosing of some agents with large pharmacokinetic variation in the noncancer setting (including antibiotics, such as aminoglycosides and vancomycin, anticonvulsants, immunosuppressant drugs, and lithium), it has not been broadly used in oncology except to minimize toxicity with high-dose methotrexate. Additional clinical trials and implementation studies will be required before this approach can be integrated into clinical practice. Dosing based on therapeutic drug monitoring and genotyping of drug-metabolizing capacity are more sophisticated and potentially more individualized or personalized approaches but are rarely available or used.

VIAL SIZES

The need to choose vial sizes for weight-based drugs is unique to this type of drug; there is nothing analogous for fixed-dose drugs. A manufacturer will know what the recommended doses are in terms of milligrams of drug per kilogram of body weight or the equivalent for BSA and then must decide how much drug to package in each vial. If the vial is too large, a large percentage of it will likely be discarded for each single use. If it is too small, many patients will require more than one vial, and significant portions of the subsequent vials may be discarded. Manufacturers can choose to produce multiple vial sizes in an effort to minimize discarded drug, but that has its own disadvantages, as each size requires its own regulatory approval, manufacturing process and validation, inventory, shipping, and recordkeeping. An added complication is that even if a medication has been given regulatory approval for multiple vial sizes, there is no guarantee that drug manufacturers will produce or that drug distributors will carry all the approved sizes.

Finding the optimal balance between too many and too few vials has been a topic of debate for researchers and policy makers in recent years. FDA does not regulate vial sizes. Rather, it approves the sizes suggested by the new drug's manufacturer, which are determined during the clinical development phase of drug development. Manufacturing, distribution, formulation, and safety are key considerations when selecting vial size (FDA, 2013).

Manufacturing and Distribution

A key issue in selecting vial sizes is whether the drug is intended to be used for an injection or infusion of a single dose of medication. Because single-dose vials contain one dose of a drug to be used one time for a single patient, they have less excess volume. They usually do not include antimicrobial preservatives to reduce the risk of vial contamination from bacteria growth and, therefore, are discarded immediately after use. Multiple-dose vials are intended to contain more than one dose of a drug and therefore do contain antimicrobial preservatives. In the United States, FDA requires drug manufacturers to add preservatives to multiple-dose vials to prevent microbial growth (FDA, 2018c). However, some markets outside the United States have raised concerns about preserved multiple-dose drugs (Biophorum, 2020). Thus, the requirements from different markets could lead to complications in the supply chain.[9] Additionally, manufacturers may consider a high fill volume to be necessary to cover all potential weight ranges of patients, but this could lead to leftover drug for lower-weight patients.

One way to reduce the amount of discarded drug for lower-weight patients is to offer multiple vial sizes for a drug. That leaves manufacturers and distributors with two big decisions: how many different sizes should be offered and what quantity of each to produce. With multiple sizes, each size must be developed, validated, and manufactured. This increases the effort and time required to bring a drug to market. In addition, managing multiple vial sizes of the same product may add complexity to manufacturing and distribution logistics, such as inventory and administrative costs. Each new vial size must be sent to regulatory agencies in multiple countries for validation and approval in order to manage a global supply chain or inventory. Furthermore, all sizes of the same product would typically have the same shelf life, but the demand may differ for different vial sizes and some vial sizes may be less likely to be used before the expiration date than others.

Formulation and Safety

The physical form in which a drug is manufactured or administered (e.g., powders or injectable or infusible solutions) is decided on in the early phases of its clinical trial. After drug development, different sectors of the biopharmaceutical supply chain come together to introduce the drug to market. The United States Pharmacopeia (USP) prepares a monograph for each drug, which is a detailed label that provides information regarding the identity, quality, purity, strength, packaging (e.g., multiple- or single-dose vials), and labeling requirements.

[9] To the committee's knowledge, there is a dearth of available publications that suggests that drugs currently contained in single-dose vials would not work well or pose safety concerns when they are mixed with antimicrobials and packaged into multiple-dose vials.

GUIDANCE FROM FEDERAL AND NONGOVERNMENTAL ORGANIZATIONS

FDA, the Centers for Medicare & Medicaid Services (CMS), and the Centers for Disease Control and Prevention (CDC) all develop regulations and guidelines that have implications for ensuring access to effective drugs, public safety, and managing federal health care spending. However, because these agencies' guidelines are not harmonized and may even be in conflict with each other, systematic efforts to reduce discarded drugs can be a challenge. In addition to the federal guidance, recommendations from scientific nongovernmental organizations that set standards aimed at ensuring drug safety (such as the USP) have enormous downstream ramifications for public spending by Medicare and private health care payers.

FDA

FDA makes regulatory decisions on how drugs can be used safely and effectively (FDA, 2018a) which can influence the cost of medications. During its review of medical products, FDA approves package size, package type terms, and discard statements as part of product labeling (FDA, 2017). Currently, however, FDA does not regulate vial sizes as part of the drug approval process. FDA has limited influence over the vial sizes that an individual manufacturer markets or over the design of the foundational clinical trials that sponsors submit as a prerequisite to obtaining regulatory approval. This also includes the oversight of clinical trials undertaken by companies that seek to obtain new drug labels or modify existing drug labels, although there are evidently some aspects of FDA oversight that clearly influence what manufacturers do. In October 2018, FDA issued guidance on selecting appropriate language for labeling injectable medical products for human use, packaged in multiple-dose, single-dose, and single-patient use containers (FDA, 2018b). Specifically, the recommendations sought to provide clarity on drug labels to help address unsafe injection practices resulting from improper use of medication vials for more than one patient.

CMS

CMS has implemented various approaches to cost containment for its health insurance programs (namely Medicare and Medicaid), including managing coverage decisions for drugs. Although CMS encourages health care providers to use drugs in the most efficient way in order to contain drug costs, it also expects providers to use drugs in a clinically appropriate manner, and this requirement leads to situations where the remainder of a single-dose vial must be discarded after administering the necessary amount of the drug to patient. In 2007, CMS introduced the JW modifier, a coding mechanism to separately report the amount of a drug used from a single-dose vial and the discarded amount when submitting claims for reimbursement. This policy was initially voluntary, but in 2017, CMS made it mandatory (CMS, 2016). A detailed discussion on reimbursement with the JW modifier is presented later in the chapter.

Currently, Medicare reimburses health care providers up to the amount of drug indicated on the vial or package label of a single-dose product, including what is discarded, and patients have cost-sharing responsibility for both the portion they receive and the portion that is discarded. Health care providers must use the smallest package size available from the manufacturer or the package size that is the closest to the patient's prescribed dosage amount (CMS, 2016).

CDC

Although CDC does not have oversight of drug availability and spending, its policies have implications for health care expenditures and drug safety. Currently, CDC guidelines call for single-dose vials to be used for one patient only (CDC, 2019). The intention is to protect patients from infectious disease outbreaks that may occur if a vial is contaminated after its first puncture and then reused. If microorganisms or contaminants enter a vial and are able to grow before its next use, the second recipient could potentially develop an infection (CDC, 2019). However, no clear evidence exists that vial sharing is responsible for any clinically significant infections. Nevertheless, CDC guidance and concerns about liability stemming from the risk of infection serve as a restraint to vial sharing.

USP

The USP is an independent, scientific, nonprofit organization that sets standards for the identity, strength, quality, and purity of medicines. These standards are based on public comments and expertise from relevant stakeholders, including patients, academics, regulatory authorities, the health care industry, and drug manufacturers (USP, 2020a). Medicines contained in single-dose vials are either given directly via injection or mixed with a solution or another drug, packaged, and labeled—a process known as *compounding*—to create a new formulation to be given to a patient as an infusion using a drug-delivery device (FDA, 2018d). As FDA does not approve compounded drugs (FDA, 2018d), the USP guidance (called "General Chapters") for compounding establishes procedures, methods, and practices that practitioners use to help ensure the quality of compounded preparations (USP, 2020b). USP General Chapter 797 specifies that after an initial puncture of a vial or once part of the contents of a vial have been extracted—generally by inserting a needle attached to a syringe—any remaining contents must be used within 1 hour unless the vial is kept in an International Organization for Standardization (ISO) 5 environment,[10] which extends the time to 6 hours (USP, 2009). In addition, USP General Chapter 1151 on injections provides guidelines to drug manufacturers on designing their products to meet the label claim and acceptable overfill to avoid excesses and deficiencies that may arise from overfills and allow for correct dosing (USP, 2012).

Current Guidance on Repackaging Single-Dose Vials

FDA, CMS, and CDC each have established guidance on the repackaging of single-dose drugs—that is, dividing the content of a single-dose vial into multiple individual doses— with varying parameters (see Figure 2-2). According to FDA (2015b), "appropriately labeled, single-dose vials that contain significantly more drug than is required for a single dose may result in the misuse of the leftover drug product." Similarly, it noted that "the need to combine several single-dose vials for a single patient dose may lead to medication errors and microbial contamination" (FDA, 2015b). FDA conveys caution but is silent on whether repackaging is allowed:

- "Single-dose vials should not contain a significant volume beyond what would be considered a usual or maximum dose for the expected use of the drug product.
- Consumers and/or health care providers should not be routinely required to use more than one vial to administer a typical single dose of the drug product."

According to CMS (2012), "it is permissible for health care personnel to administer repackaged doses derived from a single-dose vial to multiple patients, provided that each repackaged dose is used for a

---

[10] An ISO 5 environment is a primary engineering control, such as a laminar airflow workbench or compounding aseptic isolator, that allows for no more than 100 particles per cubic foot of air, which acts to minimize the chances of a vial being contaminated by environmental microorganisms (USP, 2009). A variety of classification types govern cleanroom cleanliness, but the primary system in the United States is the International Organization for Standardization (ISO). The cleanroom class is the level of cleanliness the room complies with, according to the quantity and size of particles per volume of air. The minimum standard for pharmaceutical cleanrooms is generally ISO 5.

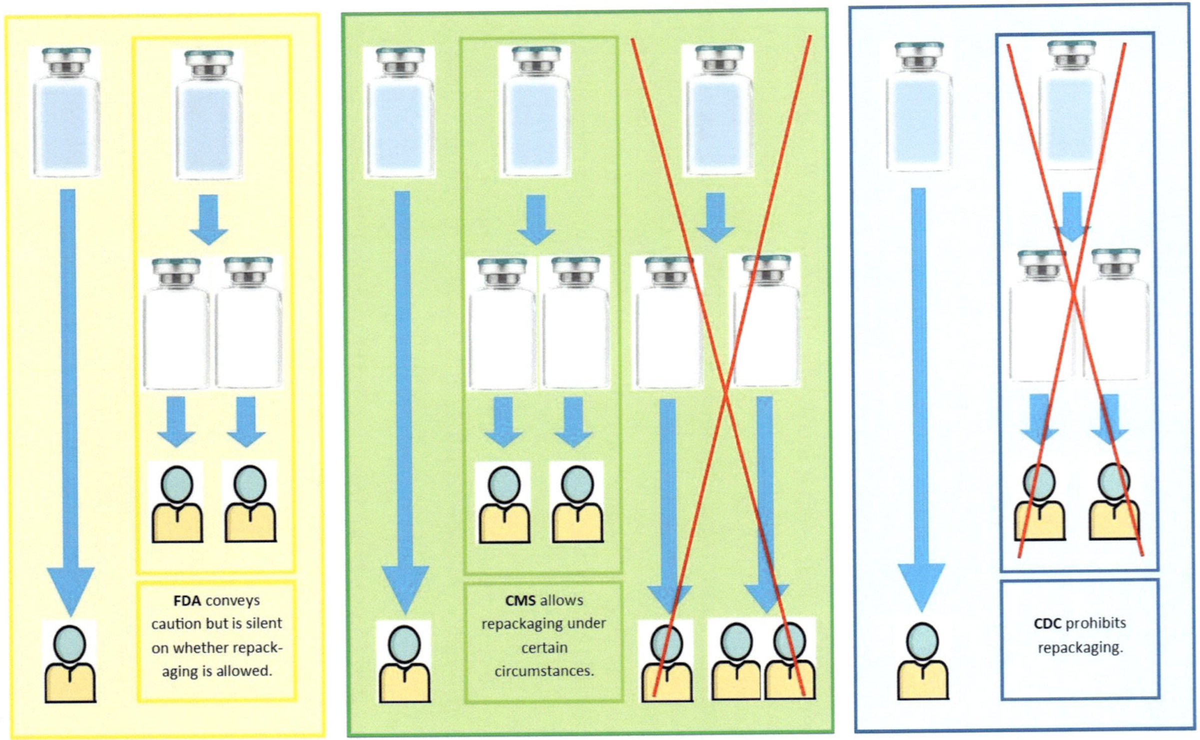

FIGURE 2-2 Comparison of FDA, CMS, and CDC guidance on the use of single-dose vials.
NOTE: CDC = Centers for Disease Control and Prevention; CMS = Centers for Medicare & Medicaid Services; FDA = U.S. Food and Drug Administration.

single patient in accordance with applicable storage and handling requirements." CMS allows repackaging under specified conditions, using qualified, trained personnel under ISO Class 5 conditions and a primary engineering control, which is used for preparing supplies for drug repackaging under a hood.

According to CDC, vials labeled as single-dose should only be used for one patient and should not be split into multiple single-use vehicles (e.g., syringes) (CDC, 2019).

Also, the USP allows for the contents of a single-dose vial to be prepared into multiple final dosage forms in either an infusion bag or syringe if all the conditions in USP General Chapter 797 are followed (USP, 2016). Some U.S. hospitals with ISO 5 facilities use vial sharing by scheduling multiple patients who are treated with the same drug to come in on the same day, a process known to some as *batching* (see Chapter 4). Because USP General Chapter 797 has an outsized influence on the extent of vial sharing, its policies have enormous downstream ramifications for public spending by Medicare and private spending by health care payers.

Repackaging single-dose vials into multiple doses creates a billing challenge for the health care system. The expectation is that a single patient is charged for the full vial, not for what was used. This could lead to the system seeking full reimbursement for one vial from each of multiple patients who shared a vial. That is, if two patients are dosed from a single-dose vial, reimbursement for its full cost could be sought from each patient or insurer—potentially at a profit for the system. There are at least two ways to avoid this incentive: produce vial sizes that are better calibrated to the average single dose or refine the reimbursement system to allow the health care system to charge partial amounts. The latter possibility is hindered by the lack of harmonization across agencies as to whether repackaging is appropriate.

CLINICIAN ACQUISITION OF AND PAYMENT FOR DRUGS

The final leg of the journey of single-dose drugs from manufacturer to patient is the administration by a physician and the associated payments for this service. Heath care providers have different arrangements with intermediaries such as distributors and pharmacy benefit managers (PBMs), and with health care payers for obtaining the drugs. The intermediaries typically handle most aspects of the drug-purchasing process on behalf of private payers, federal and state programs, employers, and other payer types.

Distributors[11] negotiate and purchase drugs directly from manufacturers at a discounted rate, and generally follow current good manufacturing practices (CGMPs) to ensure that the drugs are stored appropriately and safely.[12] They then sell the drugs to clients at a wholesale acquisition cost plus some negotiated percentage. Distributors may choose not to stock all available sizes of the same product, as this would require additional storage space, suppliers, and transportation expenses and impose a risk that the products may exceed their allowable shelf life before leaving the distribution center. PBMs negotiate contracts and drug prices with drug manufacturers and wholesalers on behalf of payers and pharmacies (NASEM, 2018; Schulman and Richman, 2018). They are significant in the distribution of specialty drugs.[13] PBMs manage drug formulary and use management strategies to define the lists of drugs that a physician can administer to a patient and receive reimbursement for based on the individual's health insurance plan (Royce et al., 2020). PBMs receive payments for their administrative services plus a portion of negotiated rebates from manufacturers (NASEM, 2018; Sood et al., 2017). Some PBMs operate their own specialty pharmacies and offer patients mail services for drugs to be sent to the physician for administration in a practice setting. Currently, many of the largest health insurance companies in the United States have PBMs (Paavola, 2019).[14]

Clinician Acquisition of Weight-Based Drugs

Traditionally, most clinician-administered drugs have been acquired and distributed by a process known as "buy and bill" (Polite et al., 2014) (see Figure 2-3), under which the health care provider is responsible for managing drug inventory at the practice setting. These health care providers acquire the drugs by purchasing from manufacturers directly or

---

[11] Three distributors—AmerisourceBergen, Cardinal Health, and McKesson—cover almost 92 percent of the market. In 2017, specialty drugs, many of which are infusible, and injectable drugs that are dispensed in weight-based, single-dose vials, accounted for more than 30 percent of full-line distributors' revenues (Deloitte, 2019).

[12] CGMPs include procedures for storing drug products under appropriate conditions of temperature, humidity, and light so that the identity, strength, quality, and purity are not affected.

[13] *Specialty drugs* is a general label for medications that are highly expensive, are complex molecularly, have limited availability or a specialized distribution network, have unique storage or shipment requirements, and are used for treating rare and complex disease indications. The pharmacies that stock and distribute these specialty drugs are referred to as *specialty pharmacies*.

[14] UnitedHealth owns both CatamaranRx and OptumRx as PBMs; Aetna now has access to CVS Caremark, the PBM of CVS Health; Anthem owns a PBM called *IngenioRx*; Cigna merged with Express Scripts; and Humana has an in-house PBM.

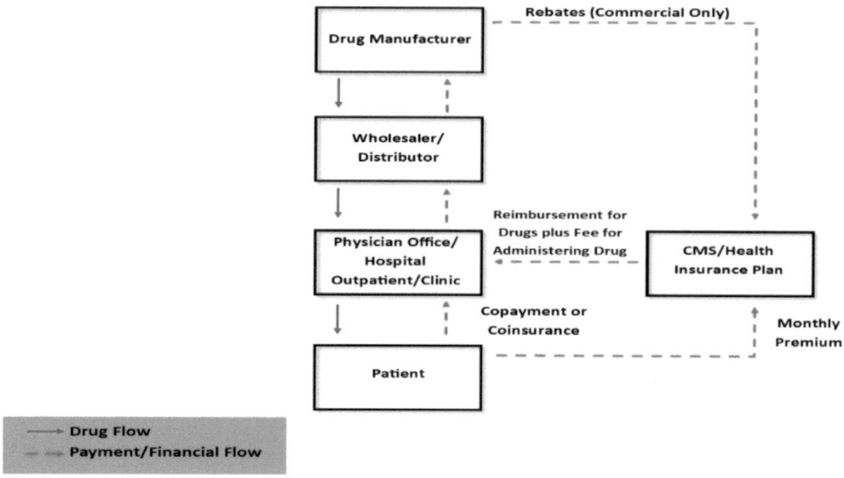

FIGURE 2-3 Flow of payments and drugs with buy and bill.
NOTE: For drugs in single-dose vials, physicians are reimbursed for the drug administration fee plus an amount for the quantity of drug that is discarded.

from intermediaries, such as wholesalers or specialty pharmacies; they then store them in their practices, administer them as needed, and submit a claim to either Medicare or the patient's health insurance. This means that the provider decides which vial sizes to buy and stock, often with no or little knowledge of the types of patients the physicians' practices and hospital outpatient departments serve. Over the past decade, buy and bill has been criticized for creating incentives for physicians to choose the drug with the higher market-based price in situations where there are therapeutic alternatives (Berndt and Newhouse, 2012).

Currently, some payers have adopted arrangements to circumvent buy and bill for physician-administered drugs that involve contracting with third-party specialty pharmacies that handle drug acquisition instead of the providers directly purchasing the drug. These alternatives are known as *white bagging* (see Figure 2-4) and *brown bagging* (see Figure 2-5).

In white bagging, heath care providers purchase patient-specific medication from a pharmacy, typically a specialty pharmacy, and the patient pays the copayment or coinsurance to the pharmacy. The pharmacy delivers the medication directly to the physician's office, hospital or clinic, and a clinician administers the drug. The payer reimburses the pharmacy. Some health care providers, particularly rural hospitals and smaller clinics, may find it advantageous to use white bagging to avoid concerns about stocking drugs that may not be used before their expiration date.

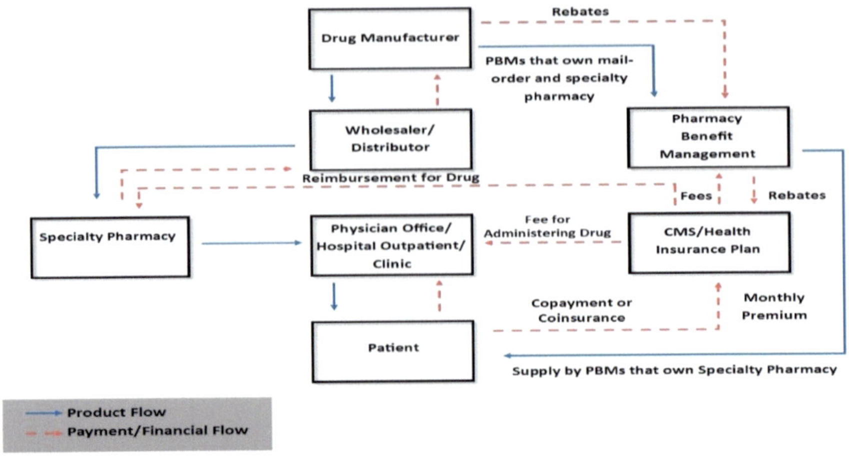

FIGURE 2-4 Flow of payments and drugs under "white bagging."
NOTES: For drugs in single-dose vials, physicians are reimbursed for the drug administration fee plus an amount for the quantity of drug that is discarded. The process reduces the opportunity for the physician office, hospital, or clinic to earn margin on the medication itself.

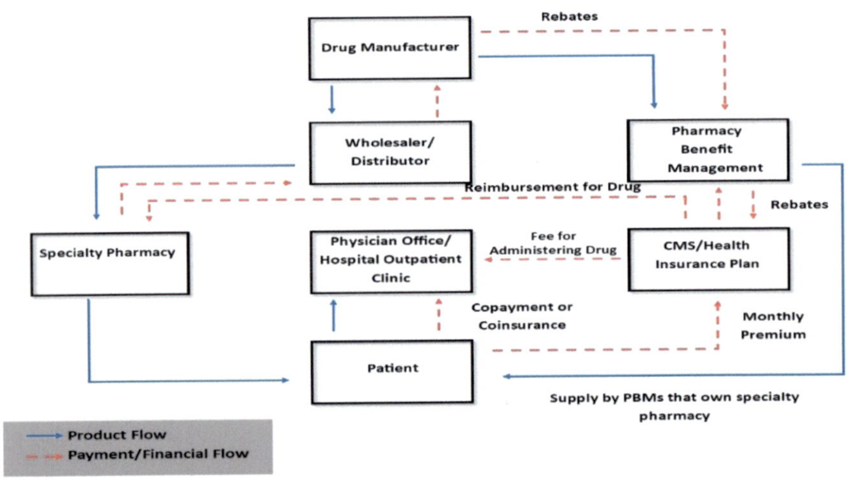

FIGURE 2-5 Flow of payments and drugs under "brown bagging."
NOTES: For drugs in single-dose vials, physicians are reimbursed for the drug administration fee plus an amount for the quantity of drug that is discarded. The process reduces the opportunity for the physician office, hospital, or clinic to earn margin on the medication itself.

Under brown bagging, the specialty pharmacy dispenses the drug directly to the patient, who transports the drug to the health care provider. Again, the physician neither buys nor bills for the drug but is paid a drug administration fee.

Both white bagging and brown bagging reduce a physician's cost for purchasing and stocking expensive medications. The physician is paid only for the professional services associated with administering the drug. However, since a drug acquired through these means can only be given to the patient for whom it was ordered, any excess in the vial must be discarded even under conditions where vial sharing may be permitted. Also, both methods may increase medication errors, may lead to delays in care, and can negatively impact patient outcomes (ASCO, 2016).

Although some commercial payers are using alternative arrangements that remove providers from the drug acquisition process, buy and bill is still the traditional method of payment for provider-administered drugs (Drug Channels, 2016).

Current Payments for Clinician Administration of Infused or Injected Drugs

The likelihood of discarding drugs is also influenced by how clinicians are reimbursed by payers. Spending on clinician-administered drugs under Medicare Part B is highly concentrated in a relatively small number of drugs (ASPE, 2020). The top 20 drugs in terms of Medicare payment amount accounted for almost 60 percent of the total Part B spending on prescription drugs in 2017 (ASPE, 2020).

As mentioned in Chapter 1, the Medicare Modernization Act of 2003 established average sales price (ASP) as the basis for Medicare Part B drug reimbursement. The ASP payment model reimburses clinicians based on the ASP plus a percentage add-on for administering the drug.[15] As a result, the ASP add-on for administration is higher for high-priced drugs than low-priced drugs. Administrative complexity is not necessarily proportional to the ASP, however. The ASP payment model was designed more than a decade ago to cover any added acquisition-related expenses for handling and storing the drugs. An unintended consequence of the current ASP payment model is that it has the potential to incentivize use of higher priced drugs because administration-related payment to clinicians increases with the price of the drug (Jacobson et al., 2010; OIG, 2012; Werble, 2017), many of which have been identified as those with the JW modifier used to indicate discarded drug from single-dose vials. (See Box 2-1 for a discussion on the JW modifier.)

---

[15] See https://www.congress.gov/bill/108th-congress/house-bill/1 (accessed September 23, 2020).

BOX 2-1
The JW Modifier

Since January 2017 the Centers for Medicare & Medicaid Services (CMS) has required health care providers to report the portion of drug from a single-dose vial that is discarded and eligible for payment under the "discarded drug policy" with a particular code called the JW modifier. Under this CMS policy, health care providers receive payment for up to the total amount of drug indicated on the vial or package label of a single-dose product, including that which is discarded, and patients have cost-sharing responsibility for both the portion they receive, and the portion that is discarded. The JW modifier can be used for any single-dose vial in which some drug is discarded, regardless of whether the drug is administered in a fixed dose or a dose based on weight.

As the analysis in Chapter 3 shows, not all providers use the JW code, and those who do use it do so inconsistently. Some have viewed this policy as providing economic incentive for wastage and hindering efficient ways to distribute or administer drugs because clinicians and hospitals can still be reimbursed whether or not the drug is actually used (Goldstein and Hirsch, 2018).

Compliance with the JW requirement would ensure that CMS is able to track the amount of drug that is discarded from single-dose vials but does not offer practical application to addressing the issue of discarded drugs. Furthermore, the JW modifier does not comprehensively capture the scope of discarded drugs. Currently, according to CMS, the modifier should not be used for drugs or biologicals administered in a rural health clinic or a federally qualified health center, claims for hospital inpatient admissions that are billed under the Inpatient Prospective Payment System, and drugs or biologicals in multi-dose vials. Additionally, in situations where the waste cannot be quantified (e.g., when multiple doses are prepared in advance), the JW modifier is not required. It is also not to be used for overfill[a] or when the actual dose of the administered drug is less than the Healthcare Common Procedure Coding System billing unit (CMS, 2016).

---

[a] For injectable drug products that are packaged in vials, biopharmaceutical manufacturers usually include a small overfill (FDA, 2015b). Because it can be difficult to completely remove all the contents of the vial, the overfill helps to ensure that appropriate doses can be withdrawn. FDA published recommendations pertaining to allowable excess volume in injectable vials in June 2015 (FDA, 2015b) that called on biopharmaceutical companies to more tightly control the amount of excess product contained in vials of injectable drugs and biologics in order to avoid excesses and deficiencies that may arise from overfills. Neither patients nor health care payers are billed for overfill, and the waste referred to in this report does not pertain to that overfill component.

For drugs in single-dose vials, Medicare pays health care providers for the quantity of drug that is administered to the patient and the quantity that is discarded, in addition to the fee for administering the drug.

Impact of Payment Policy on Patients

When patients are responsible for drug cost-sharing, their share is based on the full content of the single-dose vial even if they received just a portion of it. Traditional fee-for-service Medicare beneficiaries are responsible for up to 20 percent of the Medicare-approved amount for covered Part B prescription drugs (CMS, 2020c), and approximately 81 percent of these beneficiaries have supplemental insurance or drug coverage purchased separately, from Medicaid, or from prior employers to cover some or all of this cost (Cubanski et al., 2019). The other 19 percent of beneficiaries have no supplemental coverage and are required to pay the 20 percent coinsurance for Part B drugs out of pocket, with no cap on annual total out-of-pocket expenses. As a result, part of the cost of the discarded portion of a single-dose vial is passed along to patients, almost always without their knowledge. Although those patients with supplementary insurance are insulated from these costs, patients without it may find that their financial responsibility includes the discarded portion of the drug. Among Medicare beneficiaries with cancer, those without supplemental insurance incur substantially higher out-of-pocket costs than their counterparts with private or other supplemental coverage (Narang and Nicholas, 2017). Therefore, while the number of Medicare beneficiaries affected by this issue may be a small portion of the Medicare population, the people affected face undue burden of out-of-pocket costs.

Thus, in an era where Medicare Part B drug spending is growing faster than drug spending in other federal health care programs, the United States has a tremendous opportunity to realign incentives to encourage health care providers to make the most efficient choices for their patients and to decrease the amount of drugs discarded.

Realigning Incentives for Clinician Administration of Infused or Injected Drugs

In the past decade, proposals from the federal government—from both the U.S. Congress and the executive branch—on paying for clinician-administered drugs have focused on an array of provisions that seek to eliminate misaligned financial incentives and address the growing concerns about rising costs, quality of care, and inefficient spending. One proposal, for instance, has been to change the provider add-on percentage to a flat rate fee (MedPAC, 2015; NASEM, 2018). In other words, health care providers would no longer be reimbursed based on a percentage of the ASP of the drug dispensed. Other proposals have called for developing payment bundles for drugs and services (Werble, 2017) and for using private-sector vendors to procure, distribute, and bill Medicare for certain Medicare clinician–administered drugs (Sachs, 2018).

Under the current ASP payment model, prescribers largely determine which drugs are to be purchased, and patient cost-sharing is specified by health insurance plans. Medicare and private payers reimburse health care providers for the drugs they administer based on the drug's average sales price plus a percentage add-on for administering the drug. Uncoupling the payments from the drug average sales price and focusing the payment for clinical administration on CMS's assessment of the time and complexity of treatment administration and safety monitoring would minimize incentives for clinicians' selection and administration of more expensive drugs when alternatives are available. These payments could be made to vary somewhat based on drug categories and classes.

The Center for Medicare & Medicaid Innovation (CMMI), which is managed by CMS, has designed, implemented, and tested new health care payment models to deliver better health outcomes to Medicare beneficiaries while reducing spending. For example, indication-based pricing sets specific prices based on particular drug indications that are paid to the manufacturer according to the expected efficacy of a drug in each of its indications (Chandra and Garthwaite, 2017; CMS, 2018). The oncology care model encourages participating health care providers to improve care and lower costs through episode-based payment approaches (CMS, 2020a). CMS defines an episode as "the set of services provided to treat a clinical condition or procedure" (CMS, 2020b). The episode-based payment approach combines all the payments for services during an episode of illness—from diagnoses, procedures, and drugs furnished to a beneficiary—into a single payment.

Reimbursement by treatment episode rather than by the volume or the vial cost is a form of the episode-based model. The model's basic idea is to minimize the influence of drug-derived revenue on clinician-administered drugs, given the rapidly rising drug costs and expenditure in the Medicare Part B program. The underlying concern with discarded weight-based drugs is that payers believe that they are paying for discarded medication. One approach to addressing this issue would be to focus on efforts to reallocate unused drugs by sharing vials among multiple patients. As described later in this chapter, to the extent that these practices become widespread, drug manufacturers are likely to adjust prices of their drugs upward to reflect the fact that more patients are being treated by the same amount of a given drug. Raising drug prices combined with the costs associated with developing methods to allocate drugs to multiple patients from single-dose vials would likely not result in any actual financial savings to payers and patients. This would reflect true economic waste in the sense that those resources used to reallocate drugs would not have generated additional cost reductions to payers.

PATIENT QUALITY OF CARE

The quality of a patient's care is the most important consideration in every aspect of health care. Specifically, patients who are receiving weight-based drugs need to be able to trust that these drugs are effective and prepared under safe conditions and that medical errors in dosing will be avoided. This section examines patient safety and quality-of-care issues related to weight-based drugs, with a particular focus on the implications for small practices and rural hospitals.

Changing Roles of Health Care Providers

Peeling away all the layers of the drug manufacturing process, public policy, and health care financing, the clinician writes a prescription for a patient for whom a particular dosage of a weight-based drug is expected to treat that patient's disease or condition. Health care is regulated by professional codes of ethics and guidelines, which are set by a wide variety of professional societies. For any health care professional, the best interest of the patient should be at the core of the practice. At least three ethical principles are at the heart of the provider–patient relationship: beneficence, nonmaleficence, and respect for autonomy. Adhering to beneficence and nonmaleficence, clinicians take actions that maximize their patients' health and well-being and avoid actions that will unnecessarily harm their patients. When it comes to a drug in a single-dose vial, the goal is to maximize the likelihood that the correct dose is prescribed and the drug is delivered as directed. By its very nature, a single-dose vial is meant to minimize the risk of vial contamination. Repackaging a single-dose vial into smaller doses (dividing the contents of one vial into two or more) increases the risk of vial contamination. While the clinician may be aware that additional compound remains in the vial or enough is left behind to dose another patient, what happens to the vial and its contents is secondary to delivering the appropriate level of care to the patient being treated at that moment.

The ethical norms that ought to guide the practice of clinicians are set and monitored by oversight bodies in the form of licensing and accreditation requirements (IOM, 2000). Additional ethical norms come into play when there is an institutional stakeholder involved in purchasing, delivering, and overseeing medications.

Stewardship

Stewardship in the context of a health care system has at least two meanings. A health care system has a responsibility to care for both its patient population and the overall system that delivers the care to its patients. In the latter sense, being a good steward involves responsibly managing financial and human resources. Stewardship for health care providers in the case of the appropriate use of single-dose vials means balancing the available resources with the best interest of the patient population. This balance likely creates an incentive for some systems to minimize the amount of drug they discard. One way to do this at a health care system level would be to consider drawing multiple doses from a single-dose vial. As discussed earlier, according to the USP, CMS, and FDA, it is possible to repackage the contents of a single-dose vial if all the conditions in USP General Chapter 797 are followed (USP, 2016). The risk of contamination can be minimized, especially when a licensed pharmacist conducts repackaging (dividing a single-dose vial into more than one sterile vial). This approach would make the most sense in a large outpatient setting where multiple patients needing the same medication could be scheduled on the same day for treatment.

Accountability

The health care system is accountable to a variety of stakeholders, including its patients and the purchasers of the health care it delivers. In reference to patients, a health care system should be as transparent as possible in care delivery, including with medications. One concern is that when a single-dose vial is prescribed for a patient, the patient may be unaware that the charge will be for the full vial and not just what was used. Generally speaking, patients do not realize that some of the medication is discarded or that the cost of the discarded portion is billed to their insurance carrier or to them as direct costs in the form of copayment or coinsurance (if they have no insurance). This lack of transparency can lead to economic harm to the patient and leaves the patient out of any public policy discussion about vial size (i.e., patients might demand action if they understood the expense). However, using the single-dose vials as prescribed also minimizes the risk of contamination. Some patients may consider the additional cost acceptable to avoid the additional risk. And, of course, their willingness and ability to pay will vary with the drug's cost.

KEY FINDINGS

1. *When a dosing regimen based on body size (e.g., body surface area, weight) is used in pivotal studies as part of the drug development process, then that regimen will be approved by the U.S. Food and Drug Administration. Alternatives to weight-based dosing might be just as safe and effective, but comparison of weight-based dosing with alternative dosing is seldom done in pivotal trials.*

2. *Fixed dosing can eliminate complexities in dosing and administration of drugs, such as the need to use only parts of vials or multiple vials.*

3. *Administering medications from multiple different vial sizes may increase the risk of medication error and vial contamination.*

4. *Currently, the regulation and guidance on repackaging of drugs contained in single-dose vials, from the U.S. Food and Drug Administration, the Centers for Medicare & Medicaid Services, and the Centers for Disease Control and Prevention, are in conflict.*

5. *Medicare and other private payers reimburse health care providers for the drugs they administer based on the drug's average sales price plus a percentage add-on for administering the drug. As a result, the dollar amount of the add-on is larger for drugs with higher prices.*

6. *Health care providers receive reimbursement for the quantity of drug in single-dose vials, including that which is discarded, and patients have cost-sharing responsibility for both the portion they receive and the portion that is discarded.*

7. *Regardless of health insurance provider, patients' financial responsibility in the form of copayments and coinsurance is derived from the cost of the full vial, including any discarded portion of a vial used in their treatment. Medicare beneficiaries without supplemental private or public insurance coverage are responsible for up to a 20 percent coinsurance.*

CONCLUSIONS

1. Empirical evidence supporting the use of weight-based dosing instead of fixed dosing for injectable or infused drugs is limited.

2. The use of trials considering different dosing strategies (e.g., weight based versus fixed dose) early in the drug development process could help to determine if dosing based on a patient's body size (e.g., weight or body surface area) provides greater benefit than a fixed dose for a given therapeutic agent.

3. Regulatory guidance governing vial sharing varies among the U.S. Food and Drug Administration, the Centers for Medicare & Medicaid Services, the Centers for Disease Control and Prevention, and the United States Pharmacopeia, and thus creates ambiguity and confusion for clinicians and health care administrators, although there is limited information about the safety of vial sharing.

4. Under the current system in which drugs are produced, administered or paid for, health care providers do not have incentives that encourage the efficient use of infused or injectable drugs in single-dose vials. They receive payment for up to the amount of drug indicated on the label of a single-dose vial, including that which is discarded. This lack of incentives could discourage efforts to reduce the amount of discarded drugs.

RECOMMENDATIONS[16]

RECOMMENDATION 2-1: The U.S. Food and Drug Administration should require sponsors of pivotal trials for new or extended therapeutic indications to use fixed dosing for a given clinical indication unless safety and efficacy would be compromised. Manufacturers of products already in the market should consider conducting additional studies after approval so that these drugs can, when indicated, be converted to fixed dosing.

RECOMMENDATION 2-2: The Secretary of the U.S. Department of Health and Human Services should direct the Centers for Medicare & Medicaid Services, the U.S. Food and Drug Administration, and the Centers for Disease Control and Prevention to work with the United States Pharmacopeia and other nonfederal partners, pharmacists, and infectious disease experts to review and harmonize existing policies and guidelines on drug administration and repackaging. These policies and guidelines should be informed by the successful experiences from other industrialized countries in reducing the amounts of discarded drugs.

RECOMMENDATION 2-3: The Secretary of the U.S. Department of Health and Human Services should require the Centers for Medicare & Medicaid Services (CMS) to uncouple add-on payments to clinicians for infused or injected drugs under Medicare Part B from the drug average sales price, focusing the add-on payment instead on CMS's assessment of the time and complexity of drug management and safety monitoring.[17]

---

[16] These recommendations will be discussed fully in Chapter 6.

[17] The text in this recommendation was modified since the prepublication release of this report to improve technical accuracy of the language around payments to clinicians for infused or injected drugs under Medicare Part B.

RECOMMENDATION 2-4: The Secretary of the U.S. Department of Health and Human Services should require the Center for Medicare & Medicaid Innovation to design and evaluate new payment models that reimburse health care providers by treatment episode, rather than by the volume or cost of a drug vial. Findings from the demonstrations should be disseminated widely to other relevant federal agencies, private payers, purchasers, clinicians, and consumers.

REFERENCES

Ahmed, S., Z. Zhou, J. Zhou, and S.-Q. Chen. 2016. Pharmacogenomics of drug metabolizing enzymes and transporters: Relevance to precision medicine. *Genomics, Proteomics & Bioinformatics* 14(5):298–313.

ASCO (American Society of Clinical Oncology). 2016. *"Brown bagging" and "white bagging" of chemotherapy drugs.* https://www.asco.org/sites/new-www.asco.org/files/content-files/advocacy-and-policy/documents/2016-ASCO-Brown-Bagging-White-Bagging-Brief.pdf (accessed August 17, 2020).

ASPE (Office of the Assistant Secretary for Planning and Evaluation). 2020. *Report to Congress: Prescription drug pricing.* May 2020. https://aspe.hhs.gov/system/files/aspe-files/263451/2020-drug-pricing-report-congress-final.pdf (accessed October 27, 2020).

Belle, D. J., and H. Singh. 2008. Genetic factors in drug metabolism. *American Family Physician* 77(11):1553–1560.

Berndt, E. R., and J. P. Newhouse. 2012. Pricing and reimbursement in U.S. pharmaceutical markets. In P. M. Danzon and S. Nicholson (eds.), *Oxford handbook of the economics of the biopharmaceutical industry.* Cambridge, UK: Oxford University Press. Pp. 201–265.

Biophorum. 2020. *Written testimony of Biophorum to the Committee on Implications of Discarded Weight-Based Drugs.* September 2020.

Brunton, L., B. Knollmann, and R. Hilal-Dandan. 2017. *Goodman & Gilman's: The pharmacological basis of therapeutics, 13th edition.* New York: McGraw-Hill.

CDC (Centers for Disease Control and Prevention). 2019. *Questions about single-dose/single-use vials.* https://www.cdc.gov/injectionsafety/providers/provider_faqs_singlevials.html (accessed August 5, 2020).

Chandra, A., and C. Garthwaite. 2017. The economics of indication-based drug pricing. *New England Journal of Medicine* 377(2):103–106.

Charani, E., M. Gharbi, M. Hickson, S. Othman, A. Alfituri, G. Frost, and A. Holmes. 2015. Lack of weight recording in patients being administered narrow therapeutic index antibiotics: A prospective cross-sectional study. *BMJ Open* 5(4):e006092.

CMS (Centers for Medicare & Medicaid Services). 2012. *Safe use of single dose/single use medications to prevent healthcare-associated infections.* https://www.cms.gov/Medicare/Provider-Enrollment-and-Certification/SurveyCertificationGenInfo/Downloads/Survey-and-Cert-Letter-12-35.pdf (accessed August 5, 2020).

CMS. 2016. Medicare program JW modifier: Drug/biological amount discarded/not administered to any patient frequently asked questions. https://www.cms.gov/medicare/medicare-fee-for-service-payment/hospitaloutpatientpps/downloads/jw-modifier-faqs.pdf (August 7, 2020).

CMS. 2018. *Indication-based formulary design beginning in contract year (CY) 2020.* https://www.cms.gov/newsroom/fact-sheets/indication-based-formulary-design-beginning-contract-year-cy-2020 (accessed August 7, 2020).

CMS. 2020a. *Oncology care first model: Informal request for information.* https://innovation.cms.gov/files/x/ocf-informalrfi.pdf (accessed August 31, 2020).

CMS. 2020b. *Oncology care model.* https://innovation.cms.gov/innovation-models/oncology-care (accessed August 31, 2020).

CMS. 2020c. *Prescription drugs (outpatient).* https://www.medicare.gov/coverage/prescription-drugs-outpatient (accessed October 1, 2020).

Cubanski, J., T. Neuman, S. True, and M. Freed. 2019. *What's the latest on Medicare drug price negotiations?* http://files.kff.org/attachment/Issue-Brief-Whats-the-Latest-on-Medicare-Drug-Price-Negotiations (accessed August 31, 2020).

Deloitte. 2019. *The role of distributors in the US health care industry: 2019 report.* https://www2.deloitte.com/content/dam/Deloitte/us/Documents/life-sciences-health-care/us-hda-role-of-distributors-in-the-us-health-care-industry.pdf (accessed August 17, 2020).

Drug Channels. 2016. *Follow the vial: The buy-and-bill system for distribution and reimbursement of provider-administered outpatient drugs.* https://www.drugchannels.net/2016/10/follow-vial-buy-and-bill-system-for.html (accessed August 17, 2020).

FDA (U.S. Food and Drug Administration). 2005. *Guidance for industry estimating the maximum safe starting dose in initial clinical trials for therapeutics in adult healthy volunteers.* https://www.fda.gov/regulatory-information/search-fda-guidance-documents/estimating-maximum-safe-starting-dose-initial-clinical-trials-therapeutics-adult-healthy-volunteers (accessed October 28, 2020).

FDA. 2013. *Guidance for industry safety considerations for container labels and carton labeling design to minimize medication errors.* https://www.fda.gov/files/drugs/published/Safety-Considerations-for-Container-Labels-and-Carton-Labeling-Design-to-Minimize-Medication-Errors.pdf (accessed October 28, 2020).

FDA. 2014. *KEYTRUDA (pembrolizumab) for injection, for intravenous use Initial U.S. Approval: 2014.* https://www.accessdata.fda.gov/drugsatfda_docs/label/2014/125514lbl.pdf (accessed November 11, 2020).

FDA. 2015a. *Drug development and review definitions.* https://www.fda.gov/drugs/investigational-new-drug-ind-application/drug-development-and-review-definitions (accessed August 17, 2020).

FDA. 2015b. *Allowable excess volume and labeled vial fill size in injectable drug and biological products: Guidance for industry.* https://www.fda.gov/media/88138/download (accessed August 5, 2020).

FDA. 2017. *Repackaging of certain human drug products by pharmacies and outsourcing facilities: Guidance for industry.* https://www.fda.gov/media/90978/download (accessed August 5, 2020).

FDA. 2018a. *Current good manufacturing practice (CGMP) regulations.* https://www.fda.gov/drugs/pharmaceutical-quality-resources/current-good-manufacturing-practice-cgmp-regulations (accessed August 17, 2020).

FDA. 2018b. *Facts about the current good manufacturing practices (CGMPS).* https://www.fda.gov/drugs/pharmaceutical-quality-resources/facts-about-current-good-manufacturing-practices-cgmps (accessed August 17, 2020).

FDA. 2018c. *Selection of the appropriate package type terms and recommendations for labeling injectable medical products packaged in multiple-dose, single-dose, and single-patient-use containers for human use guidance for industry.* https://www.fda.gov/regulatory-information/search-fda-guidance-documents/selection-appropriate-package-type-terms-and-recommendations-labeling-injectable-medical-products (accessed August 17, 2020).

FDA. 2018d. *Step 3: Clinical research.* https://www.fda.gov/patients/drug-development-process/step-3-clinical-research (accessed August 17, 2020).

FDA. 2020. FDA approves new dosing regimen for pembrolizumab. https://www.fda.gov/drugs/drug-approvals-and-databases/fda-approves-new-dosing-regimen-pembrolizumab (accessed August 17, 2020).

Goldstein, D. A., and A. Hirsch. 2018. A policy that encourages wastage of expensive medications—the JW modifier. *JAMA Oncology* 4(2):155–156.

Hall, E., J. Zhang, E. J. Kim, G. Hwang, G. Chu, S. Bhatia, and S. Reddy. 2020. Economics of alternative dosing strategies for pembrolizumab and nivolumab at a single academic cancer center. *Cancer Medicine* 9(6):2106–2112.

Hendrikx, J. J. M. A., J. B. A. G. Haanen, E. E. Voest, J. H. M. Schellens, A. D. R. Huitema, and J. H. Beijnen. 2017. Fixed dosing of monoclonal antibodies in oncology. *The Oncologist* 22(10):1212–1221.

IOM (Institute of Medicine). 2000. *To err is human: Building a safer health system*. Washington, DC: National Academy Press.

Jacobson, M., C. C. Earle, M. Price, and J. P. Newhouse. 2010. How Medicare's payment cuts for cancer chemotherapy drugs changed patterns of treatment. *Health Affairs* 29(7):1391–1399.

Kaestner, S. A., and G. J. Sewell. 2007. Chemotherapy dosing part I: Scientific basis for current practice and use of body surface area. *Clinical Oncology* 19(1):23–37.

Markman, M. 2005. "Flat-fixed dosing" of chemotherapy: A concept whose time has come? *Current Oncology Reports* 7(1):1–2.

Mathijssen, R. H., F. A. de Jong, W. J. Loos, J. M. van der Bol, J. Verweij, and A. Sparreboom. 2007. Flat-fixed dosing versus body surface area based dosing of anticancer drugs in adults: Does it make a difference? *The Oncologist* 12(8):913–923.

MedPAC (Medicare Payment Advisory Commission). 2015. Chapter 3: *Part B drug payment policy issues*. http://www.medpac.gov/docs/default-source/reports/chapter-3-part-b-drug-payment-policy-issues-june-2015-report-.pdf (accessed August 31, 2020).

Musuamba, F. T., E. Manolis, N. Holford, S. Cheung, L. E. Friberg, K. Ogungbenro, M. Posch, J. Yates, S. Berry, N. Thomas, S. Corriol-Rohou, B. Bornkamp, F. Bretz, A. C. Hooker, P. H. Van der Graaf, J. F. Standing, J. Hay, S. Cole, V. Gigante, K. Karlsson, T. Dumortier, N. Benda, F. Serone, S. Das, A. Brochot, F. Ehmann, R. Hemmings, and I. S. Rusten. 2017. Advanced methods for dose and regimen finding during drug development: Summary of the EMA/EFPIA workshop on dose finding (London 4–5 December 2014). *CPT: Pharmacometrics & Systems Pharmacology* 6(7):418–429.

Narang, A. K., and L. H. Nicholas. 2017. Out-of-pocket spending and financial burden among Medicare beneficiaries with cancer. *JAMA Oncology* 3(6):757–765.

NASEM (National Academies of Sciences, Engineering, and Medicine). 2018. *Making medicines affordable: A national imperative*. Washington, DC: The National Academies Press.

OIG (Office of Inspector General). 2012. *Least costly alternative policies: impact on prostate cancer drugs covered under Medicare Part B* (OEI-12-12-00210). https://oig.hhs.gov/oei/reports/oei-12-12-00210.pdf (accessed January 27, 2021).

Paavola, A. 2019. *The top insurers all have PBMs: Here's who they are*. https://www.beckershospitalreview.com/pharmacy/the-top-insurers-all-have-pbms-here-s-who-they-are.html (accessed August 17, 2020).

Pai, M. P. 2012. Drug dosing based on weight and body surface area: Mathematical assumptions and limitations in obese adults. *Pharmacotherapy* 32(9):856–868.

Pan, S., L. Zhu, M. Chen, P. Xia, and Q. Zhou. 2016. Weight-based dosing in medication use: What should we know? *Patient Preference and Adherence* 10:549–560.

Polite, B. N., J. C. Ward, J. V. Cox, R. F. Morton, J. Hennessy, R. D. Page, and R. M. Conti. 2014. Payment for oncolytics in the United States: A history of buy and bill and proposals for reform. *Journal of Oncology Practice* 10(6):357–362.

Royce, T. J., C. Schenkel, K. Kirkwood, L. Levit, K. Levit, and S. Kircher. 2020. Impact of pharmacy benefit managers on oncology practices and patients. *JCO Oncology Practice* 16(5):276–284.

Sachs, R. 2018. Administration outlines plan to lower pharmaceutical prices in Medicare Part B. *Health Affairs Blog* 26.

Schulman, K. A., and B. D. Richman. 2018. The evolving pharmaceutical benefits market. *JAMA* 319(22):2269–2270.

Selvan, V. A., S. H. Calvert, G. Cavell, E. Glucksman, M. Kerins, and J. Gonzalez. 2007. Weight-based N-acetylcysteine dosing chart to minimise the risk of calculation errors in prescribing and preparing N-acetylcysteine infusions for adults presenting with paracetamol overdose in the emergency department. *Emergency Medicine Journal* 24(7):482–484.

Sood, N., K. Van Nuys. T. Shih, and D. Goldman. 2017. *Follow the money: The flow of funds in the pharmaceutical distribution system.* https://www.healthaffairs.org/do/10.1377/hblog20170613.060557/full (accessed August 5, 2020).

Tamargo, J., J.-Y. Le Heuzey, and P. Mabo. 2015. Narrow therapeutic index drugs: A clinical pharmacological consideration to flecainide. *European Journal of Clinical Pharmacology* 71(5):549–567.

USP (United States Pharmacopeia). 2009. *Chapter <797> pharmaceutical compounding: Sterile preparations* https://www.usp.org/compounding/general-chapter-797 (accessed August 5, 2020).

USP. 2012. *Chapter <1151> pharmaceutical dosage forms.* https://www.drugfuture.com/pharmacopoeia/usp35/PDF/0765-0784%20%5B1151%5D%20Pharmaceutical%20Dosage%20Forms.pdf (accessed August 5, 2020).

USP. 2016. *Briefing injections.* https://www.usp.org/sites/default/files/usp/document/harmonization/gen-method/q08_pf_31_1_2005.pdf (accessed December 9, 2020).

USP. 2020a. *About USP.* https://www.usp.org/about (accessed August 5, 2020).

USP. 2020b. *USP compounding standards.* https://www.usp.org/compounding-standards-overview (accessed August 5, 2020).

Werble, C. 2017. *Medicare Part B.* Health Affairs Health Policy Brief. https://www.healthaffairs.org/do/10.1377/hpb20171008.000171/full (accessed November 20, 2020).

3

Scope of Discarded Drugs from Single-Dose Vials

The costs and payments for discarded medications from single-dose vials and how that cost and payment should be estimated have been a subject of much debate in recent years. In the 2019 *Part B Discarded Drug Units Report*, the Centers for Medicare & Medicaid Services (CMS) reported that in 2018 it had paid $725 million (or 2.1 percent of the total Medicare allowed amount for Part B drugs) for discarded medications administered in hospital outpatient clinics and physicians' offices (CMS, 2019). CMS obtained that estimate by aggregating all Part B drug claims with the JW modifier associated with the claims. This calculation assumed that providers consistently use the mandatory JW modifier, which has not been verified empirically.[1] Another analysis in 2016 estimated the money spent on discarded drugs in single-dose vials of cancer medications to be $1.8 billion (Bach et al., 2016).[2] Furthermore, the analysis suggested that the amount of money spent on discarded medications by public and private health care payers swelled to $2.8 billion when physician and hospital markups were included in the estimate (Bach et al., 2016).

In addition to its formal Statement of Task, CMS charged this committee to use "available data sources to quantify the amount of *waste* associated with single-dose injectable drugs and biologics in billing units and/or proportion of available vial sizes and calculate the associated dollar amounts." Both federal and private entities have attempted to

[1] The analysis excluded beneficiaries in the Medicare Advantage program, which represents approximately 36 percent of the Medicare population (Freed et al., 2020).

[2] This study was conducted before the policy mandating the JW modifier.

assign a dollar value to these unused portions. To more fully understand the extent of health care costs—to the Medicare program, private health care payers, and patients—that arise from billing for discarded drugs and biologicals from single-dose vials, the committee commissioned two analyses of these costs. The researchers who conducted the analyses had a data-use agreement with CMS and IBM MarketScan that allowed them to conduct this work using the 2017 and 2018 Medicare and MarketScan databases.[3] The focus of these analyses are not to assess the economic value of the discarded drug but rather to get a sense of the amount of drugs that are being discarded and to identify any inefficiencies in the current system of tracking the amount of discarded drugs yearly.

A committee subgroup was tasked with working directly with the researchers and guiding the analyses. The researchers made presentations to the full committee during closed deliberations and received guidance from the full committee, and the committee validated the findings from the analyses, which are summarized below. Further details from the commissioned analyses are provided in Appendix B.

ANALYSIS OF MEDICARE SPENDING ON DISCARDED DRUGS[4]

The first commissioned analysis examined Medicare claims that used the JW modifier code,[5] examining how much of total Medicare spending they represent; examined patterns in the claims using the JW modifier code and whether those claims accurately reflected the amount spent each year by Medicare on discarded drugs; and explored compliance with the JW modifier. The analysis was performed using a 20 percent random sample

---

[3] The Medicare and MarketScan data are publicly available to any researcher, but a licensing fee and a data-use agreement with CMS are required to obtain the Medicare data, and a license fee and agreement are also required to obtain MarketScan data from IBM Watson Health. The issue of discarded drugs is not unique to Medicare and Medicare beneficiaries. Some private health insurance companies tend to follow CMS policy on discarded drugs as well, which is why the committee commissioned analyses that used both Medicare and MarketScan data.

[4] This section draws on analyses commissioned by the Committee on Implications of Discarded Weight-Based Drugs on "The extent of health care costs—to the Medicare program, to private health care payers, and to patients—that arise from billing for discarded drugs and biologicals from single-dose vials" by Aditi P. Sen, Ph.D. (assistant professor, Department of Health Policy and Management, Johns Hopkins Bloomberg School of Public Health) and Hui Zhao, Ph.D. (associate professor, Department of Health Services Research, Division of Cancer Prevention and Population Sciences, The University of Texas MD Anderson Center).

[5] As described in Chapter 2, the JW modifier is the mechanism through which health care providers can bill and be reimbursed for the discarded portion of a single-dose vial in a way that formally documents the amount of drug that was discarded. The modifier can be used for any single-dose vial in which some drug is discarded, regardless of whether the drug is administered in a fixed dose or a dose based on weight.

of traditional fee-for-service Medicare outpatient and carrier claims from 2017 to 2018, with a focus on discarded drugs and biologicals. Claims for which Medicare was not the primary payer were excluded. The researchers specifically included the 77 drugs with the highest total allowed amounts[6] in the *2018 Medicare Part B Discarded Drug Units Report* (CMS, 2019). The discarded drugs and the associated spending were identified based on claim lines with the JW modifier code. According to that CMS report, the total Part B spending in 2018 on all drugs with discarded amounts was $34.8 billion; the report estimated that $725 million was spent on the discarded portions of these drugs. The 77 drugs in the committee's commissioned analysis accounted for 83 percent of the total spending and 92 percent of the spending on the discarded portions. Of the 77 drugs, 34 are administered with weight-based dosing, 12 use body surface area (BSA)-based dosing, and 31 are given in fixed doses.[7] (See Box 3-1 for a brief explanation of why certain fixed-dose drugs in single-dose vials could have portions discarded.) As discussed in previous chapters, in this report, *weight-based drugs* refers to drugs that are dosed either by weight or by BSA. Therefore, for the purposes of these analyses, weight- and BSA-based drugs are both described as *weight based*.

Using the data from the Medicare claims, two types of analyses were performed. One was a general analysis of the use of the JW modifier for the 77 drugs, considered jointly and individually. The other looked at variations among physicians in their use of the JW modifier. The findings were then used to provide an estimate of the total nominal cost of discarded drugs—that is, the amount of dollars represented by the discarded drugs under the assumption that the discarded drugs could be valued at the same per-unit cost as unused drugs in single-use vials—and that number was compared with the total cost indicated by the JW modifier.

Claims-Level Analysis

Of the claims involving the 77 drugs with the greatest total Medicare payouts for discarded amounts, a surprisingly small percentage actually

---

[6] Total Medicare allowed amount for a given Part B drug includes the amount Medicare pays, the deductible and coinsurance amounts that the beneficiary is responsible for, and any amounts that a third party is responsible for.

[7] The classification of the dosing regimen of the drugs for our analysis was abstracted by reviewing the package insert provided by FDA for each of the 77 drugs in the *Medicare Part B Discarded Drug Units* report included in the analysis. The insert includes prescription drug labeling resources, which lists detailed information on dosage and administration. If the dosage is based on patients' weight or BSA, then we define the drug as weight based; otherwise, it is classified as fixed dose. The 31 drugs classified as fixed dose had the JW modifier associated with them.

BOX 3-1
Why Some Fixed-Dose Drugs in Single-Dose Vials Have Discarded Portions

Sometimes portions of fixed-dose drugs in single-dose vials are discarded. This can happen, for instance, when a drug is used to treat more than one disease or condition and the amount used for each indication differs. Consider, for example, onabotulinumtoxinA, which is available in 50-unit (1.25 mL), 100-unit, or 200-unit single-dose vials.[a] For treating overactive bladder, a fixed dose of 100 units is used, but for chronic migraine, the fixed dose is 155 units, and for axillary hyperhidrosis, the fixed dose is 50 units per axilla. If a patient is being treated for overactive bladder and the clinician has either the 50-unit or 100-unit vial available, no drug would be discarded. However, if only the 200-unit vial was available, 100 units of medication would be discarded. To treat a migraine patient with the recommended 155 units, 45 units would be discarded regardless of whether the treatment used a 200-unit vial or some combination of the 50-unit and 100-unit vials. This situation is common with certain other fixed-dose drugs. Thus, depending on the indication, different amounts of a fixed-dose drug from a single-dose vial could be administered to a patient, and the remaining drug would have to be discarded.

[a] See https://www.accessdata.fda.gov/drugsatfda_docs/label/2017/103000s5302lbl.pdf (accessed July 25, 2020).

included the JW modifier (i.e., differentiated the discarded amount from the administered amount when submitting their claims). In 2017, 16.2 percent of the claims had the JW modifier, and in 2018, 16.9 percent did. This finding suggests low compliance[8] with the CMS mandate. The percentage of claims with the JW modifier was substantially higher among weight-based (26.9 percent in 2018) than fixed-dose (1.4 percent) drugs (see Table 3-1).[9] JW modifier use was relatively concentrated, with 21 of the 77 drugs having over 25 percent of claims with the JW modifier. The drugs with the highest percentage of claims with the JW modifier fell into the following classes: oncology (30 drugs, with an average of 18 percent of claims having the JW modifier), rheumatology (12 drugs, 16 percent), and respiratory (6 drugs, 5 percent).

Looking only at the weight-based drugs in the Medicare sample, the researchers found that the use of the JW modifier was not prevalent. The

[8] The level of compliance is determined by whether the JW modifier was used at all and not related to the specific amount of discarded drug recorded.

[9] MarketScan analysis will be discussed later in this chapter.

TABLE 3-1 Percentage of Claims with the JW Modifier by Drug Dosage Category in Medicare and MarketScan Databases, 2017 and 2018

	Medicare		MarketScan	
	Weight-based (n=46)	Fixed-dose (n=31)	Weight-based (n=46)	Fixed-dose (n=31)
Percentage of claims with the JW modifier, 2017	25.3	1.9	5.83	1.49
Percentage of claims with the JW modifier, 2018	26.9	1.4	6.74	2.16

committee recognizes that in some cases, the JW modifier would not be reported because the entire contents of the vial were used in the treatment of a single patient, or there was no discarded drug because the vial may have been shared between patients in accordance with United States Pharmacopeia guidelines. However, approximately half of the drugs had the JW modifier coded in fewer than 10 percent of the claims; in 2018 the JW modifier was used in more than 10 percent of the claims for only 24 of the 46 drugs (see Figure 3-1, blue bars).

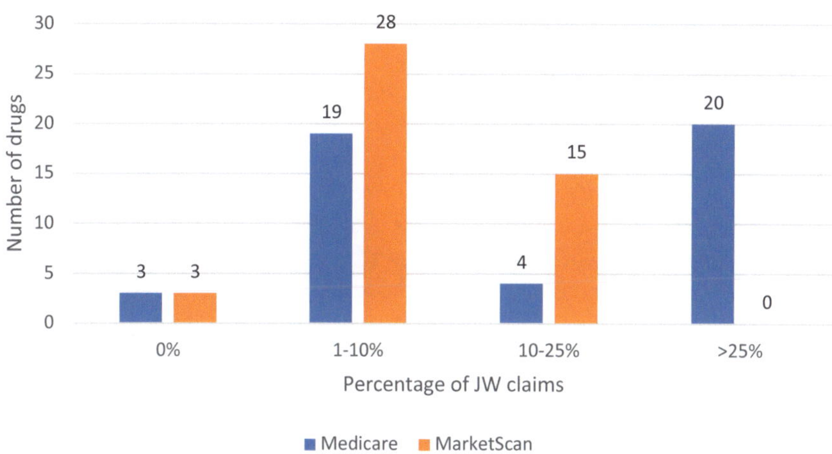

FIGURE 3-1 Percentage of JW claims among 46 weight-based drugs in Medicare and MarketScan data in 2018.

Provider-Level Analysis

The second part of the Medicare analysis examined variations in use of the JW modifier according to a number of physician-related factors that might be correlated with discarding more or less drug or with compliance with the JW modifier coding requirements. There was a very low correlation between total spending on a drug and percentage of claims with the JW modifier.[10] Among those drugs in the sample for which at least 1 percent of claims used the JW modifier (40 of 77 drugs), there were few consistent patterns or substantial differences in terms of use of the modifier across regions,[11] nor did the use of the JW modifier in urban versus rural areas follow any sort of consistent pattern.[12]

The analysis also examined the role of provider volume in terms of using the JW modifier. The rates of use were similar between health care providers with above and below the median number of claims for a particular drug and also between health care providers in the bottom 25th and top 25th percentiles of claims for that drug.[13]

The only consistent pattern identified across drugs was higher use of the JW modifier in physician office settings relative to hospital outpatient departments.[14] Across the 40 drugs in the sample with at least 1 percent of claims with the JW modifier, a higher percentage of physician office settings used it for a given drug than hospital outpatient departments did. A number of factors may be driving this pattern, including billing practices in offices versus outpatient departments and differences in payment systems.

Given that use of the mandated JW modifier is a provider-level behavior, the committee explored whether noncompliance might be concentrated among a subset of providers and existing estimates of the amount of discarded drugs might thus be underestimates due to noncompliance. The commissioned analysis does demonstrate that a substantial proportion of physicians who prescribe drugs in the sample never use the JW modifier. In the 20 percent Medicare fee-for-service sample, a total of 163,646 health care providers had at least one claim for 1 of the 77 drugs. To look for a pattern of noncompliance, analyses were limited to health care providers with more than 10 claims, and among the 42,034 health care providers who had made at least 10 claims for at least one of the 77 drugs, 28,457 (67.7 percent) never used the JW modifier at all (see Figure 3-2).

---

[10] For more detailed data, see Figure B-4 in Appendix B.
[11] For more detailed data, see Figure B-5 in Appendix B.
[12] For more detailed data, see Figure B-6 in Appendix B.
[13] For more detailed data, see Figure B-7 in Appendix B.
[14] For more detailed data, see Figure B-8 in Appendix B.

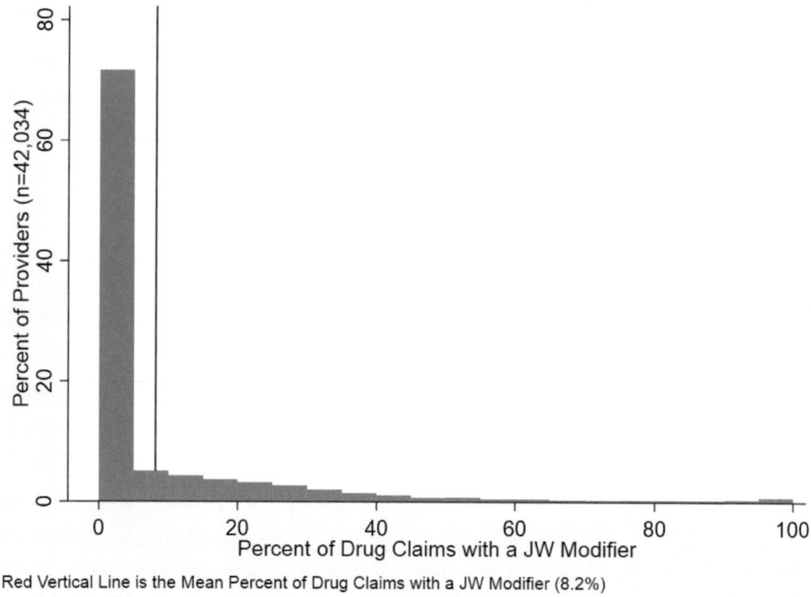

FIGURE 3-2 Provider-level use of the JW modifier, 2018.
NOTES: Analysis restricted to health care providers who had more than 10 claims for at least one of the top 77 drugs. The drugs included in the analysis were the 77 drugs (Healthcare Common Procedure Coding System codes) with the highest total allowed amounts in the *2018 Medicare Part B Discarded Drug Units Report*. Analysis conducted using the 20 percent Medicare sample.

Patient–Drug Pairs Level of Analysis

Not only is there significant variation among physicians in the use of the JW modifier, but many individual physicians are themselves not consistent about it, even when filing claims for the same patient on the same drug. It is reasonable to assume that if a certain amount of a particular drug for a particular patient is marked with the JW modifier on one occasion, the modifier is likely appropriate in all instances of that patient receiving that drug within a relatively short period, since the dosage is based on weight or body size. Yet, an analysis of the five drugs with the greatest Medicare spending on claims with the JW modifier (Table 3-2, left panel)[15] found that the modifier was used inconsistently in a significant number of cases where a patient was given the same drug on multiple

[15] MarketScan data on the right panel will be discussed later in this chapter.

TABLE 3-2 Health Care Provider Use of the JW Modifier for a Patient–Drug Combination in Medicare and MarketScan Data, 2018

	Medicare JW Modifier Compliance (%)			MarketScan JW Modifier Compliance (%)		
Generic Name	Full	No	Partial	Full	No	Partial
Bortezomib	60.8	16.5	22.7	17.2	64.2	18.6
Trastuzumab	36.0	28.6	35.5	3.9	78.9	17.3
Romiplostim	37.2	19.2	43.7	7.5	71.2	21.3
Paclitaxel Protein-Bound	49.2	26.6	24.2	14.1	71.8	14.1
Carfilzomib	40.7	21.3	38.0	22.8	66.7	10.5

NOTES: Top five drugs in terms of spending on claims with the JW modifier. Patient–drug combinations with at least two observations. Trastuzumab use refers to reference biologic only.

occasions. For example, in 23 percent of patient–drug combinations with bortezomib, the JW modifier was used in some but not all cases, while the percentage of inconsistent usage was 44 percent for romiplostim.

Similarly, the analysis found substantial variation in how likely health care providers were to use the JW modifier from one drug to another. This part of the analysis was restricted to the 25 drugs in the sample with at least 10 percent claims with the JW modifier and was also restricted to providers with at least 11 claims for the drug. The number of providers included in the analysis varied widely according to the particular drug, from 9 providers with at least 11 claims for ipilimumab to close to 2,000 providers with at least 11 claims for onabotulinumtoxinA. In this sample, the percentage of providers who never used the JW modifier varied across drugs, from 8 percent of those administering brentuximab vedotin to 70 percent of those administering infliximab.[16]

The large percentages of health care providers with more than 11 claims who used the modifier in some cases but not others present clear evidence that providers are using the JW modifier inconsistently from one drug to another. Equally important, over two-thirds of the providers with 11 or more claims for at least one of the 77 drugs never used the JW modifier at all.

Estimated Costs of Discarded Drugs

Given the evidence that many physicians are not using the JW modifier at all and that those who do apply it are doing so inconsistently from

[16] For more detailed data, see Figure B-3 in Appendix B.

one drug to the next and even from one treatment to the next for the same patient, it seems clear that a significant percentage of discarded drugs are never reported via the JW modifier and so the estimates of the total cost of discarded drugs based on the aggregation of Medicare claims with the JW modifier are likely to be significantly low. To get a sense of just how low, the analysis examined the top five drugs in terms of spending associated with claims with the JW modifier and estimated the amount of unreported spending on discarded drugs.

First, the researchers calculated a patient drug–specific ratio of JW-associated spending to total spending for claims with the JW modifier and then applied that ratio to calculate additional potential spending for observed encounters where the patient received the drug but there was no claim with the JW modifier.[17] The total spending on discarded drug as a percentage of total spending for the drug was 9–27 percent without accounting for the amount of unreported spending. After including the estimated amount of unreported spending using the approach described above, the total spending on discarded drug was 11–28 percent of total spending. Even after including the estimated unreported spending, these figures are likely an underestimation because it is not possible to project potential spending for patient–drug combinations where the JW modifier was never used, which accounts for a sizable percentage of patient–drug combinations.

Another approach to estimate costs of discarded drugs is to include only health care providers who used the JW modifier. Excluding health care providers who never used the JW modifier, the average percentage of claims with the JW modifier was 59 percent and the average spending on these claims was 11 percent of total spending among the 25 drugs with at least 10 percent of claims with the modifier in 2018. These levels compare to 50 percent and 10 percent, respectively, when all providers (including those who never used the modifier) are included in the analysis.[18] In some drugs (e.g., omalizumab), the difference in the percentage spending on JW claims could be as large as 50 percent (i.e., 10.3 percent versus 6.3 percent).

The committee recognizes the limitations of this analysis. The researchers who performed the analysis did not have access to durable medical equipment claims, for example, and these would likely capture additional amounts of discarded drugs (e.g., for products delivered via inhalers). Also, data from Medicare Advantage, which now covers approximately 36 percent of Medicare beneficiaries, were not included (Freed et al., 2020). Finally, although the Medicare claims data suggest that beneficiaries are likely to be responsible for coinsurance on discarded

[17] For more detailed data, see Table B-1 in Appendix B.

[18] For more detailed data, see Table B-2 in Appendix B.

products, it was not possible to precisely capture beneficiary out-of-pocket spending due to the unavailability of data on supplemental private or public coverage (e.g., Medigap), which commonly covers cost-sharing for some patients.

ANALYSIS OF PRIVATE PAYERS' SPENDING ON DISCARDED DRUGS

The second set of analyses examined the use of the JW modifier among privately insured patients and estimated the cost associated with discarded drugs for both patients with private health care and their payers.

Claims-Level Analysis

To get a sense of how often the JW modifier is used in claims on private insurance policies, the researchers used IBM MarketScan research databases to identify it in both the Commercial Claims and Encounters and Medicare Supplemental databases from 2017 to 2018. Using the same 77 drugs selected in the above Medicare analysis, they examined the patterns of JW code use in the private insurance market, identifying claims for the 77 drugs from MarketScan data by using the Healthcare Common Procedure Coding System codes for those drugs.

Out of more than 4 million claims in 2017 and 2018, the overall percentage with the JW modifier was very low—just 3.62 percent. Fifteen of the 77 drugs had zero JW claims. Among the 62 drugs with at least one JW claim, less than 1 percent to 22.2 percent, for azacitidine (J9025), had the JW modifier in the claims. As Table 3-1 shows, the use of the JW modifier in weight-based drugs in the MarketScan database was substantially lower than the pattern found in the Medicare analysis, as not all private insurance claims require health care providers to use it. When limiting the analysis to only weight-based drugs, findings from the analysis of MarketScan data showed that the use of the JW modifier was even more concentrated than the pattern observed in Medicare data. As Figure 3-1 shows, only 15 of the 46 weight-based drugs had more than 10 percent of the claims submitted using the JW modifier.

The JW modifier was used more often for weight-based than fixed-dose drugs, and oncology, neuromuscular, and rheumatology drugs were the most likely to have it. The JW modifier was more prevalent among patients with Medicare supplemental insurance than among those with private, employment-based insurance, those who received treatment in 2018 versus 2017, and those who resided in the South.

Patient–Drug Pairs Level Analysis

Although the MarketScan data did not allow for the sorts of physician-to-physician comparisons that were described above from Medicare data, it was possible to carry out an analysis with patient–drug pairs to gain insight into how consistently the JW modifier is used in claims on private insurance. The researchers categorized modifier compliance into three levels: none, partial, and full. The analysis used the same top five drugs as in the analysis of Medicare fee-for-service claims data; Table 3-2 shows the pattern of compliance based on patient–drug pairs in the MarketScan data. For patients with Medicare, the range of full compliance for these five was 36–60 percent. The corresponding JW compliance in MarketScan data was much lower, 3.9–22.8 percent.

Out of the 62 drugs with at least one JW claim, 25 drugs had more than 5 percent of JW claims at the patient–drug pair level; azacidine had the highest JW compliance rate, about 42 percent combined partial and full compliance.[19]

Estimated Costs of Discarded Drugs

Working from the MarketScan data, the researchers calculated the costs of discarded drugs as reflected in the JW modifier filings. They observed that 18 drugs had discarded amounts with a total cost greater than $1 million. The discarded amount for these 18 drugs accounted for about 89 percent of the $80.6 million total cost for the discarded amounts of all 77 drugs in MarketScan data.

The $80.6 million figure was calculated using claims with the JW modifier. However, private payers grossly underused the JW modifier.[20] The researchers imputed the potential additional spending on discarded drugs using the same approach described in the Medicare analysis by applying a patient drug–specific ratio to the partially compliant group. The researchers found that using the approach employed by CMS, discarded drugs accounted for 0.81 percent of total insurance payment on the above 18 drugs. However, this percentage was based on the underused JW modifier. When the potential additional spending imputed from the partially compliant group was included, the percentage of total insurance payment on discarded drugs increased to 1.6 percent.[21] This analysis again demonstrated the underestimation of costs associated with discarded drugs when the calculation relied on the JW modifier.

---

[19] See Table B-3 in Appendix B.
[20] See Table B-3 in Appendix B.
[21] See Table B-4 in Appendix B.

The analyses of both the Medicare and MarketScan claims data demonstrated the inadequacy of relying solely on the JW modifier to estimate costs associated with discarded drugs because the current billing practice largely does not adhere to the CMS discarded drug policy. To better understand the financial impact of discarded drugs, the researchers conducted an additional analysis that used patients' actual weight and height to determine the discarded percentage of their drugs.

In the MarketScan data, a subset of patients participated in the Health Risk Assessment (HRA) survey. The HRA data include self-reported weight, and height information. From the 77 Part B drugs, 45 weight-based drugs were found in the claims of patients who responded to the HRA survey. The researchers abstracted the recommended dosage and vial size for a drug to treat a specific disease based on IBM Micromedex and collected the claims of these 45 drugs from the 2017 MarketScan data. Then they linked the HRA data with the drug claims to select patients with known weight/height as a study cohort of 4,688 patients.[22] They computed the discarded drug units by subtracting patients' treatment drug units from the full vial sizes and calculated the percentage of the discarded drug units by dividing the discarded units over the full vial sizes. Then, they multiplied the percentage of discarded drug units with the total net pay or out-of-pocket cost for the discarded drug amount for payers and for patients.

The researchers then limited the analyses to drugs with more than 10 claims for each drug (38 drugs). The analysis included the mean, minimum, and maximum discarded percentage for each drug.[23] The mean discarded percentage ranged from less than 1 percent to close to 40 percent. Variations in patients' weight or BSA resulted in a noticeable range between minimum and maximum percentages for some drugs. The within-drug variation in the discarded percentage highlights the challenges of adhering to the JW modifier mandate, as providers will need to make the calculation for each patient based on weight at the time of treatment, which can fluctuate from one chemotherapy administration to another. It also raises a question whether payers will have sufficient real-time biometric data to verify the information submitted in claims with the JW modifier.

The researchers analyzed payment variables from claims data to estimate the financial burden of discarded drugs for private payers and patients. On average, private insurance paid $36,652 per patient on weight-based drugs, and of this amount, $2,992 (8.2 percent) was spent on discarded drugs. The mean out-of-pocket cost was $1,043, and of this,

[22] See Figure B-1 in Appendix B.
[23] See Figure B-2 in Appendix B.

$78 (7.5 percent) was spent on discarded drugs. Although the average out-of-pocket cost for discarded drugs was moderate, a small subset of patients disproportionately bore the financial burden, especially those enrolled in high-deductible plans. For these patients, the top 10 percent paid more than $380 for discarded drugs, whereas for patients not in high-deductible plans, the top 10 percent paid more than $260. A recent survey on the economic well-being of U.S. households reported that 4 in 10 adults could not cover an unexpected expense of $400 (Board of Governors of the Federal Reserve System, 2018). Using $400 as the benchmark value, this analysis found that approximately 10 percent of patients with high-deductible plans paid more than that on discarded drugs versus 4 percent for those who did not enroll in high-deductible plans.

LIMITATIONS

The committee recognizes two major limitations of these analyses and other estimates of the payments for discarded drugs produced by other researchers. First, the information from the JW modifier is insufficient to provide accurate estimates of the amounts of drugs that are discarded. Any estimate that depends on data from the JW modifier will be an underestimate because of the noncompliance with the CMS discarded drug policy, and the resulting data may not be representative. Second, the estimates are only nominal values that are based on the assumption that every ounce in a vial has an equal value and that the value of an ounce administered to treat a patient is equal to the value of an ounce of drug that is discarded. The calculations do not reflect the reality of the excess costs to patients and the system because of the factors that go into determining the price of drugs and how they are paid for. Chapter 5 explicitly challenges the assumption underlying the calculations and addresses the economics of discarded drugs using the committee's analytical construct.

KEY FINDINGS

1. *Not all health care providers use the JW modifier, and among those health care providers that use the modifier, the JW modifier is not reported consistently, even though it has been required by the Centers for Medicare & Medicaid Services since January 2017.*

2. *Current estimates on the payments for discarded drugs produce nominal values that do not accurately capture the economic value of discarded drugs because the estimates are based on the assumption that every ounce in a vial has an equal value and that the value of an ounce administered to treat a*

patient is equal to the value of an ounce of drug that is discarded, which in reality is not the case.

CONCLUSIONS

1. Currently, attempting to estimate a single value for the cost of discarded drugs from single-dose vials to the Medicare program using the JW modifier would be incomplete and underestimated because the modifier is underused by health care providers and the resulting data may not be representative. Also, information on discarded drugs from Medicare Advantage plans and other commercial insurance plans are currently not available.

2. The use of the JW modifier as a basis for data collection and measurement of the amount of discarded drugs from single-dose vials has no current practical application to addressing the issue of discarded drugs.

RECOMMENDATION[24]

RECOMMENDATION 3-1: While the current Medicare Part B drug reimbursement system is in place, the Centers for Medicare & Medicaid Services should discontinue the use of the JW modifier.

REFERENCES

Bach, P. B., R. M. Conti, R. J. Muller, G. C. Schnorr, and L. B. Saltz. 2016. Overspending driven by oversized single dose vials of cancer drugs. *BMJ* 352(352):i788.

Board of Governors of the Federal Reserve System. 2018. *Report on the economic well-being of U.S. households in 2017.* https://www.federalreserve.gov/publications/files/2017-report-economic-well-being-us-households-201805.pdf (accessed October 1, 2020).

CMS (Centers for Medicare & Medicaid Services). 2019. *Medicare Part B discarded drug units report.* https://www.cms.gov/research-statistics-data-systems/cms-drug-spending/medicare-part-b-discarded-drug-units-report (accessed August 7, 2020).

Freed, M., A. Damico, and T. Neuman. 2020. *A dozen facts about Medicare Advantage in 2020.* Kaiser Family Foundation. https://www.kff.org/medicare/issue-brief/a-dozen-facts-about-medicare-advantage-in-2020 (accessed October 13, 2020).

[24] This recommendation will be discussed fully in Chapter 6.

4

Efforts to Reduce Discarded Weight-Based Drugs

A variety of institutions and organizations, from Congress to hospitals and even individual clinicians, have sought to address the issue of discarded portions of weight-based drugs from single-dose vials. With significant portions of drug discarded each year, there has been pressure from various quarters to address the issue and, in particular, to find ways to minimize the amount of discarded drugs. This chapter provides an overview of these efforts, beginning with those undertaken by Congress and followed by policies adopted by professional organizations and approaches implemented by various health care providers.

U.S. CONGRESS

No overarching federal policy, strategy, or consensus currently exists on how to reduce the amount of discarded drugs that result from weight-based dosing of medicines contained in single-dose vials. However, actions by Congress have focused attention on specific aspects of this issue.

Several versions of draft congressional bills introduced in the 115th Congress (2017–2018) and the 116th Congress (2019–2020) that focused on discarded drug related to single-dose vials have proposed rebates from manufacturers to be directed to health care providers and payers for discarded drug amounts. Box 4-1 presents a summary of some of these bills. Most bills, however, did not propose rebates directed to patients, who would continue to have cost-sharing responsibilities for the cost of discarded drugs that were not used in their care. As discussed in previous

BOX 4-1
Select Draft Bills Focused on Waste Related to Single-Use Drug Vials

S. 2042—Reducing Drug Waste Act of 2017 and H.R. 6142—Reducing Drug Waste Act of 2018: Both would require the U.S. Food and Drug Administration and the Centers for Medicare & Medicaid Services to develop a joint action plan to reduce drug waste and better manage costs with respect to drug vial sizes and other drug-delivery systems.

S. 551—REFUND Act of 2019 and H.R. 4178—REFUND Act of 2019: This would require manufacturers of certain single-dose vial drugs payable under Part B of the Medicare program to provide rebates with respect to discarded amounts of such drugs.

S. 4199—Prescription Drug Pricing Reduction Act of 2020: First introduced in 2019, this would require manufacturers to refund the amount of payment made to providers for unused amounts of certain single-dose drugs that exceed a minimum threshold. The Secretary of Health and Human Services (HHS) would be required to report to the manufacturer the number of units of refundable drugs that were discarded, as identified by the JW modifier that the billing provider included on the claim form. The Secretary of HHS would impose a civil monetary penalty on a manufacturer that fails to pay a required refund.

chapters, Medicare beneficiaries without supplemental private or public health insurance coverage are responsible for up to a 20 percent coinsurance of the cost of drugs used in their treatment, including any discarded portion of a vial.

Based on the committee's assessment, it is not feasible to use rebates for discarded drugs to recoup significant funds that could be spent on other health care services, so manufacturer rebates for unused drug are unlikely to achieve the intended aim. Also, given the variety of ways that drugs are priced and reimbursed, a rebate system for clinician-administered drugs is likely to be quite complex. However, if the rebates that have been proposed in legislation are implemented, the committee asserts that patients need to be included in those rebates.

PROFESSIONAL ORGANIZATIONS

As the costs of expensive infusible and injectable drugs and biologics continue to rise, research and professional organizations have called for developing and adopting innovative solutions to reduce the amount of discarded drugs or increase efficiency in dispensing such drugs.

The American Society of Clinical Oncology (ASCO), a leading professional organization, has urged the Centers for Medicare & Medicaid Services (CMS) to consider better ways to identify the sources and costs of discarded chemotherapy drugs. The organization has called for such data to be made public and encouraged private payers to consider similar strategies (ASCO, 2018). ASCO, the U.S. Oncology Network, and the Hematology/Oncology Pharmacy Association (HOPA) have encouraged clinicians to adopt clinical practices such as dose rounding, dose capping, or dose banding (discussed later in this chapter). These practices are intended to reduce the amount of drug discarded when single-dose vials are used, while ensuring patient safety. HOPA has called on the relevant regulatory agencies to reconcile regulatory policies governing sterile compounding and on pharmaceutical manufacturers to increase the availability of medications in multi-dose vial formulations (HOPA, 2019). (See Box 4-2 for more on multi-dose formulations.)

The American Society of Health-System Pharmacists (ASHP), an organization that represents pharmacists who serve as care providers in acute and ambulatory care settings, has taken a position on the availability and

BOX 4-2
Multi-Dose Formulations

Multi-dose vials are intended to contain more than one dose of a drug, and they allow health care providers to treat more than one person from a content of a single vial. Multi-dose vials typically contain antimicrobial preservatives to prevent microbial growth but can still be contaminated if safe injection practices are not followed. Multi-dose vials have several benefits, including potentially more efficient use of the vial contents. For example, consider the initial distribution of the coronavirus vaccine from Pfizer. The vaccine is produced in multi-dose vials with a certain amount of overfill, as approved by the U.S. Food and Drug Administration (FDA). Because of this overfill and the ability to use the vial multiple times, emerging evidence indicates that health care providers are able to use the contents of one vial for more people than originally thought.[a] Therefore, less drug is discarded, as health care providers are able to maximize the use of the vial contents. Given that the vaccine is a scarce resource, if the excess drug were not able to be used, many more individuals would not be able to promptly receive this vaccine. While most of the drugs covered in this report are not scarce resources, this example highlights how multi-dose vials can reduce discarded drugs and maximize use of a vial's contents.

[a] FDA says Pfizer vaccine vials hold extra doses, expanding supply.
SOURCE: *Politico*, 2020.

use of appropriate vial sizes, advocating that pharmaceutical manufacturers provide vial sizes that reduce the amount of drug discarded and enhance safety. Additionally, ASHP has called on regulators, manufacturers, and other health care providers to collaborate to develop best practices on the safe use of single-dose vials (ASHP, 2019).

CLINICAL PRACTICES

Because of the rapidly increasing number of specialty medications coming to the market in single-dose vials (Lotvin et al., 2014; Watanabe et al., 2018), health systems and health care providers are being increasingly challenged to address the issues that these medications raise. These are not low-stakes considerations, given that the acquisition price and reimbursement amount for these medications can markedly affect a clinical practice's finances. Furthermore, clinicians and health care systems are increasingly burdened with making decisions about approaches to reduce the amount of medications they discard.

This section explores the various mechanisms and approaches that clinicians, physician offices, hospitals, and clinics currently employ to reduce the amount of discarded drugs and examines the consequences for health systems. Many clinicians, for example, have embraced strategies that several Organisation for Economic Co-operation and Development (OECD) countries currently use, although these are not yet well established in the United States; these strategies include vial sharing, drug vial optimization, closed-system drug transfer devices (CSTDs), dose banding, dose rounding, and dose capping, or a combination of these approaches. It is important to recognize that implementing these strategies requires a certain amount of health care worker time to plan and perform.

Vial Sharing

One suggested approach to dealing with the issue of discarded drugs is to discontinue the one vial per patient approach. To illustrate how this approach can decrease the amount of discarded drugs, Figure 4-1 shows the sort of situation that occurs in today's medical practices, with three patients who are receiving the anticancer drug bortezomib from single-dose vials, with each patient getting a different dosage and no vial sharing possible. The bortezomib comes in 3.5-mg vials. Patient 1 receives a dose of 2.45 mg (70 percent of a vial), with the remainder discarded. Patient 2 requires 50 percent of the vial, with the remainder discarded. And Patient 3 receives 60 percent of the vial, so 40 percent of the vial is discarded. This means that for the three patients, 30 percent of one vial plus 50 percent of a second vial plus 40 percent of a third vial—or 120 percent of a single vial's contents—would be discarded.

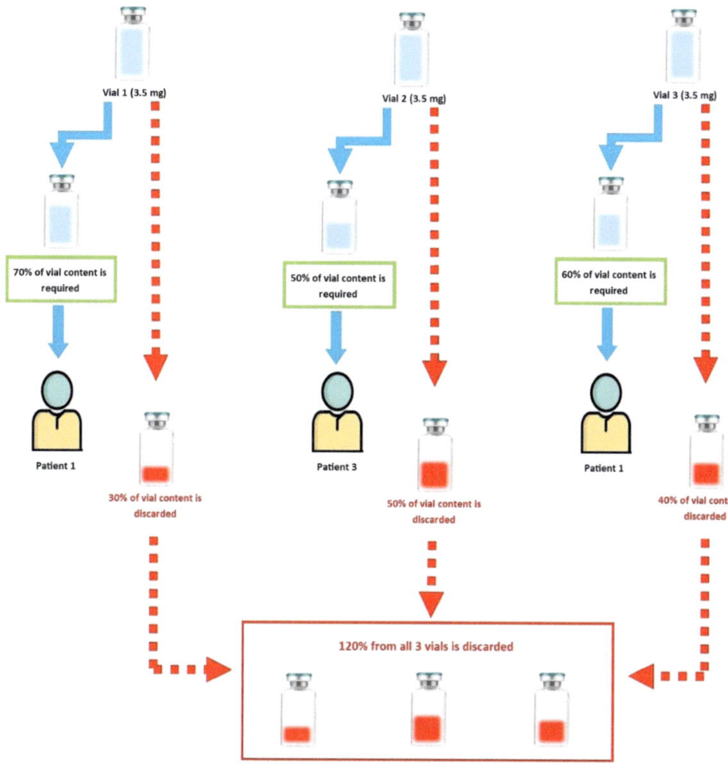

FIGURE 4-1 A representation of three patients requiring different dosages of a drug in a single-dose vial with no vial sharing possible and the amount of drug discarded.

NOTES: This example is not intended to calculate the optimal vial sizes needed but to show how vial sharing occurs among different patients with different dosage requirements once the vials are already available. It should be noted that, generally speaking, a vial's contents are not given directly to a patient but rather are removed and compounded to generate the preparation that the patient receives, but that additional step does not affect the idea behind vial sharing.

By contrast, with vial sharing, the remainder from each vial is retained and can be used for the next patient. Thus, by sharing two vials, the total discarded amount would be 20 percent of a single vial instead of 120 percent—or an entire vial saved (see Figure 4-2).

Vial sharing presents several challenges, however. Each shared vial must be unpackaged, appropriately logged, and stored, and its sterility must be ensured for later use (Smith, 2015). Multiple patients who are treated with the same drug must be scheduled to come in on

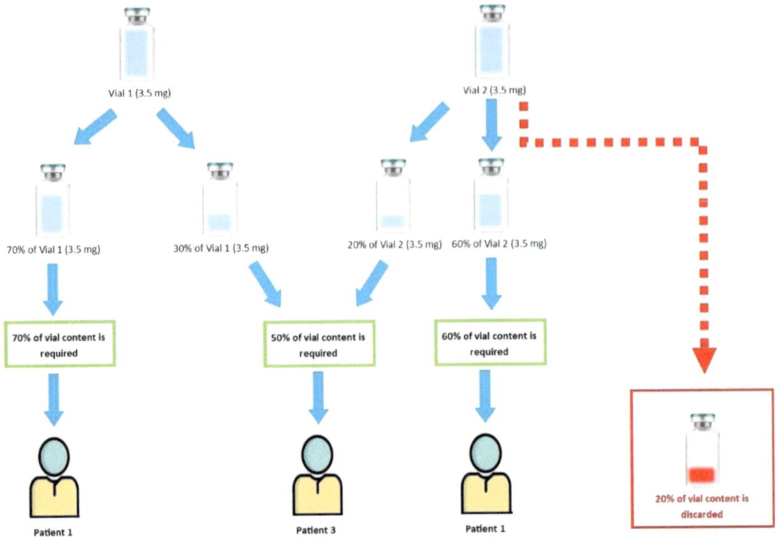

FIGURE 4-2 A representation of vial sharing among three patients requiring different dosages of a drug in a single-dose vial and the amount of drug discarded. NOTES: This example is not intended to calculate the optimal vial sizes needed but to show how vial sharing occurs among different patients with different dosage requirements once the vials are already available. It should be noted that, generally speaking, the vial's contents are not given directly to a patient but rather are removed and compounded to generate the preparation that the patient receives, but that additional step does not affect the idea behind vial sharing.

the same day, a process known to some as *batching* (discussed in detail in Box 4-3). Because two or more patients are treated from a single vial, microbial contamination is possible. Sharing a single vial can be complicated temporally, as consistently forecasting the amount of compounded product even over a few days is not simple, and the decision to puncture any individual vial will affect the usage pattern to follow. Vial sharing also demands additional attention and documentation by staff to prevent accidentally exposing multiple patients to a medication after its beyond-use date.[1] Finally, vial sharing is generally unrealistic for small clinics and facilities that do not have enough patients to make it consistently feasible.

---

[1] A beyond-use date is set by the pharmacy dispensing the drug or compounded medication and is calculated from the date or time of compounding (USP, 2019). The beyond-use date would never be later than the expiration date on the original container.

BOX 4-3
Batching

To decrease the amount of medications discarded, some clinics schedule patients receiving the same weight-based infusions for the same day in a process known as *batching*. For example, the Defense Health Agency schedules patients who need to receive the same infusion on the same day (if feasible) and adjusts the dose of the drugs, in line with guidelines from professional organizations. Given the stability rules on vials, which usually require that the contents be used within the first 6 hours after puncture (if stored under United States Pharmacopeia 797 regulations), sharing opened vials requires that multiple patients be scheduled together. In other words, by batching patients on the same day, it may be possible to minimize discarded drug by sharing vials within 6 hours. This approach functions better in larger health systems than in small, private, or rural clinics. It also demands more effort from a scheduling standpoint, and it reduces flexibility for patients, since they must generally be given fewer options for appointment times. Given that the medications are prepared in advance, batching also risks potentially magnifying the discarded medications when patients miss an appointment or a clinician reevaluates and decides to cancel the treatment for that day (Dobson et al., 2015).

Nonetheless, the advantages of vial sharing are great enough that it has come into regular use in various places around the world. It is common in Australia (Gilbar, 2020), where the Therapeutic Goods Administration—which plays a role similar to FDA in the United States—provides guidelines for the use of partial vials. The Pharmacy Board of Australia provides guidelines on assigning beyond-use dates on compounded sterile injectable products. The Society of Hospital Pharmacists of Australia supports vial sharing as long as it is carried out in specialized aseptic pharmacy facilities and follows rigorous standards of practice (Gilbar, 2020). The situation is similar in New Zealand and the United Kingdom, both of which endorse vial sharing (Gilbar, 2020). A number of studies have examined the practice of vial sharing in these and other countries and found that it reduces the amount of discarded drugs and cost of treatment (Gilbar et al., 2019; Hall et al., 2020; Rustemi et al., 2019).

Drug Vial Optimization

Certain difficulties associated with vial sharing can be ameliorated by a practice called *drug vial optimization*, which relies on extending the length of time that a drug remains sterile and stable up to as much as

7 days by using a closed-system drug transfer device (CSTD) (Amerine et al., 2019). Generally, once the sterility of the vial is breached by a puncture, the remaining drug is no longer considered safe and effective and is thus unusable. However, CSTDs make drug vial optimization possible by moving drugs from one place to another—such as from a vial into a syringe—without letting the drug or its vapor escape into the environment or introducing any contaminants into the vial or the syringe. As a result, CSTDs can ensure the stability and sterility of injectable drugs after vial puncture for much longer than the United States Pharmacopeia (USP)-specified 6 hours and safely preserve the remaining volume for later use. Manufacturers of these devices have demonstrated that the punctured vial contents remain stable and sterile for as much as a week after the beyond-use date (Gilbar et al., 2019; Juhász et al., 2016). Furthermore, CSTDs protect pharmacy personnel from exposure to those otherwise hazardous drugs (McMichael et al., 2011; Simon et al., 2016; Spivey and Connor, 2003; Wick et al., 2003). (See Box 4-4 for a detailed discussion on CSTDs.)

Though the United States was the first to implement drug vial optimization, this strategy is not supported by recent guidelines from the USP or some state boards of pharmacy (Amerine et al., 2019). Sterility is a vital criterion in drug vial optimization due to the chance of microbial contamination, which is the most common reason for policies regarding a safe duration of use (Suzuki et al., 2019). Good manufacturing practices call for the drug to be discarded after the USP's 6-hour beyond-use date (Amerine et al., 2019), which could be why current guidelines do not support drug vial optimization. However, drug vial optimization is widely accepted globally. A 2019 survey found 10 of the 12 countries surveyed had implemented this model (Suzuki et al., 2019).

Dose Banding

Dose banding is another approach to minimizing the amount of discarded drugs. In many situations there is a good deal of uncertainty with respect to optimal dosages and the risks and benefits from small or modest deviations from current dosing practices. With dose banding, doses that fall within defined ranges are set to predefined standard doses (Chatelut et al., 2012; Gilbar and Chambers, 2018; Plumridge and Sewell, 2001). Instead of doses being fixed or based on individualized weight or BSA, dose banding standardizes injectable drugs, usually in chemotherapy, into a defined set of dose ranges for patients. Each series of consecutive doses is called a *band*, with the dose to which individual doses are rounded being called the *banded dose* (Chatelut et al., 2012; Gilbar and Chambers, 2018; Plumridge and Sewell, 2001). A given drug type and class requires specific dose findings to determine the proper method for administration. This practice is well

BOX 4-4
CSTDs

Closed-system drug transfer devices (CSTDs) are systems that include multiple components that are used in various combinations when moving a drug from one container to another. To transfer a drug from the vial into a syringe, for instance, the "protector" is attached to the vial and the "injector" is attached to the syringe. The protector and the injector are then screwed together, creating an airtight seal—specifically, between two membranes, one at the edge of the protector and one at the edge of the injector, which are pressed tightly together. To transfer the drug, the plunger of the syringe is pressed, which pushes the air out of the syringe and into an expansion chamber on the protector. Next, the plunger is pulled back, which pulls the drug out of the vial into the syringe and simultaneously pulls air out of the expansion chamber to replace the drug in the vial. The drug removed from the vial is replaced with an equal amount of air, but the contents of the vial are not exposed to the external environment, and nothing from the vial escapes into the environment (Becton, Dickinson and Company, 2020; McMichael et al., 2011).

A number of studies have found CSTDs to be effective in preventing drugs or drug vapor from escaping while transferring the drug, thus offering an extra layer of protection to health care workers who handle these often toxic drugs (McMichael et al., 2011; Simon et al., 2016; Spivey and Connor, 2003). CSTDs have also been shown to be effective in preventing various microorganisms from contaminating the inside of a vial even when large amounts of the microorganisms were present on the outside of the system (De Prijck et al., 2008; McMichael et al., 2011).

By using CSTDs to extract partial contents from a single-dose drug vial, clinicians might be able to safely use the remaining contents for up to 7 days after the initial puncture, thus sharply decreasing the amount of discarded drugs—and, potentially, saving a significant percentage of the cost of the drugs (Gilbar et al., 2019). The savings assume that the resulting reduction in the volume of drugs purchased by the hospital did not affect the unit price of those drugs, which is certainly true for a single hospital. But if the nation's health care system as a whole adopted this practice, this may not hold under the current system in which drugs are developed, administered, or paid for in the United States. Indeed, a study in one hospital of nearly two dozen types of cancer drugs in single-use vials found that a CSTD saved the hospital more than $96,000 over the 50 days of the study, implying an annual savings of more than $700,000 in that one institution (Edwards et al., 2013).

established in clinical settings in the United Kingdom and several other developed countries but not in the United States (Guinto and Szabatura, 2013; Oswald, 2016; Plumridge and Sewell, 2001).

To implement this method, any health care system would need a comprehensive systematic effort to identify suitable drugs and regimens and determine the potential impact on health care systems and patient care, and valid dose-banding tables would need to be defined (Guinto and Szabatura, 2013). A few studies have shown that dose banding can reduce discarded drugs and medical errors and also preparation time (Chatelut et al., 2012; Fahey et al., 2020). However, it may be inappropriate for certain drugs or some patient populations, such as pediatric patients or significantly obese or underweight patients (Guinto and Szabatura, 2013). If a band is narrow, it may not matter, but if there is major variation in dose, the risk is that some patients could receive excess drug and others could receive insufficient treatment (Huertas et al., 2015). Small or modest deviations from current dosage practices to the banded dosage amounts may not have significant therapeutic effects but could significantly reduce the volume of drugs classified as discarded; however, this may be a result of increasing the total volume of drugs administered (in the case of upward rounding).

Dose Rounding and Dose Capping

Similar to dose banding, dose rounding is a method that either increases or decreases a prescribed dose to the nearest whole vial strength available. Simplifying a dose amount lowers medical error. This strategy has been found to be most effective when multiple vial sizes are available and rounding gives a difference no greater than plus or minus 5 percent for cytotoxic agents or plus or minus 10 percent for monoclonal antibodies[2] (Gilbar and Chambers, 2018). Implementing this method more widely could reduce the amount of discarded drug, medical errors during drug preparation, the clinical burden of documenting the unused drug and the cost of proper disposal of discarded drugs (Fahrenbruch et al., 2018). A recent analysis suggested that within 1 year, approximately $3.6 million was saved from rounding doses for 24 frequently used high-cost oncology medications (Dela Pena et al., 2020). A majority of these drugs were also among the top drugs with JW claims used to indicate discarded drug from single-dose vials. Following guidelines by HOPA, the researchers automatically adjusted up or down to the nearest full vial any dose of the drugs calculated to be within 10 percent of the nearest vial size. Within 1 year, the researchers observed that 10,200 doses of the selected drugs were administered, and half of these doses were rounded to the nearest vial size leading to some savings. Although health care providers see the

[2] Monoclonal antibodies are laboratory-produced molecules engineered to serve as substitute antibodies that can restore, enhance, or mimic the immune system's attack on cancer cells. They are designed to bind to antigens that are generally more on the surface of cancer cells than healthy cells.

potential for dose rounding to reduce discarded drugs, the degree to which the strategy is currently used in the United States is unknown.

Dose capping is a variant of dose rounding that is specifically designed to increase patient safety in obese populations. This extension acknowledges the concern that providing an obese patient with the recommended dose according to weight or body size can lead to an overdose because body composition is quite different from that of a nonobese patient of the same weight (Lyman, 2011). As U.S. obesity rates continue to rise, the need for proper guidance concerning optimal dosing in obese patients with cancer will only grow. The need for clarity has prompted ASCO to develop evidence-based clinical practice guidelines on appropriate chemotherapy dosing for obese adult patients with cancer (Lyman, 2011). ASCO has recommended that several agents be capped based on the dose that was used in clinical trials (Griggs et al., 2012).

Some have criticized these alternative dosing strategies because they may lead to patients receiving more or less drug than needed (Chatelut et al., 2012; Pouliquen et al., 2011). Another critique that several speakers at the committee's public sessions discussed is that these alternative strategies may not actually reduce spending, even though they do reduce the amount of discarded drugs, given how clinician-administered drugs are paid for in the United States. Also, as with dose banding, dose rounding may be inappropriate for some patient populations, such as pediatric patients. However, clinicians provide pediatric information regarding a primary set of recommended rounding tolerances for commonly prescribed drugs for e-prescribing (Johnson et al., 2011). Some centers may avoid dose rounding for pediatric patients or patients under a designated weight because of its ineffectiveness for amounts that are consistently much smaller than a vial's volume (Fahrenbruch et al., 2018).

Table 4-1 provides an example of how costs and wastage can vary with different dosing protocols and three different patient weights using an FDA-approved drug labeled for single use and available in three sizes.

U.S. DEPARTMENT OF HEALTH AND HUMAN SERVICES PARTNERSHIPS WITH FEDERAL AND NONFEDERAL PARTNERS

The U.S. Department of Health and Human Services (HHS) has an opportunity to effectively coordinate and collaborate with other federal agencies and nonfederal partners to identify and develop technological systems that allow single-dose vials to be used safely across multiple patients. Over the past decade, HHS has partnered with other government agencies, private organizations, and public entities to address diverse health-related issues, including developing strategies for effective solutions to address and mitigate the public health impact of diseases

TABLE 4-1 Costs Associated with Dose Rounding Versus Dosing Based on Weight Corrections

	60-kg Patient	75-kg Patient	100-kg Patient
Required dose given FDA label with 70 mg/m^2 per week as the appropriate dose	121 mg/week	134 mg/week	154 mg/week
Number of 60-mg vials	2	2	2
Number of 30-mg vials	0	1	1
Number of 10-mg vials	1	0	1
Amount discarded	9 mg	16 mg	6 mg
Total weekly cost of drug	$5,066	$5,846	$6,235
Cost of discarded drug not used for patient	$351	$624	$234
Percentage of cost of discarded drug/ total cost	7%	11%	4%
Dose rounding	120 mg/week	130 mg/week	150 mg/week
Percentage of total exact dose with dose rounding	99%	97%	97%
Total weekly cost of drug with dose rounding	$4,615	$5,222	$6,001

NOTES: The price of the drug ($38.97 per mg) was obtained from CMS's July 2020 average sales price (ASP) pricing file (https://www.cms.gov/apps/ama/license.asp?file=https%3A//www.cms.gov/files/zip/july-2020-asp-pricing-file.zip [accessed July 25, 2020]). The percentage add-on to the ASP as drug administration fees may not be exact due to rounding.

and strategies to improve patient care and health outcomes through the efficient and effective use of data.

An example is the HHS partnership to facilitate the rapid deployment of prefilled syringes for quick response to widespread health emergencies. The Rapid Aseptic Packaging of Injectable Drugs (RAPID) will enable the Strategic National Stockpile to rapidly fill and finish hundreds of millions of syringes to respond quickly and efficiently to widespread health emergencies (HHS, 2020). The RAPID consortium will identify and use technologies that eliminate the inefficiencies and difficulties of drawing medicines from glass vials to ensure that drugs are available to patients when needed.

Another example is the Accelerating COVID-19 Therapeutic Interventions and Vaccines partnership, which has brought together several agencies within HHS, including the Biomedical Advanced Research and Development Authority, the Centers for Disease Control and Prevention, and FDA, other federal agencies, including the U.S. Department of Defense and the U.S. Department of Veterans Affairs, representatives from nonprofits, including the Foundation for the National Institutes of Health, more than a dozen biopharmaceutical companies, and an international partner, the European Medicines Agency. The stated purpose of the partnership is to "develop an international strategy for a coordinated research response to the COVID-19 pandemic" (NIH, 2020). The partnership will develop a coordinated research strategy for prioritizing and allow for harmonizing and sharing preclinical evaluation methods to speed the development of the most promising treatments and vaccine.

Such effective relationships between HHS and other federal and nonfederal partners would create opportunities for developing promising and innovative systems that allow single-dose vials to be used safely across multiple patients.

INTEGRATED HEALTH CARE DELIVERY SYSTEMS, TRADITIONAL FEE-FOR-SERVICE SYSTEMS, AND THE UNDERSERVED

Different health care providers may have different incentives and barriers for reducing discarded drugs. Integrated health care delivery systems may have direct incentives to decrease the amount of discarded drugs from single-dose vials. In these systems, health care providers may be motivated to "save costs" by applying vial-sharing mechanisms or some other clinical practices for patients to reduce discarded drugs through a cumbersome and expensive process that they still view as cost-effective. Additionally, clinicians in integrated health care delivery systems are typically not paid based on the price of the drug they administer. But a traditional fee-for-service system, where health care providers are reimbursed up to the amount of drug indicated on the vial or package label of a single-dose product, including what is discarded, may have less motivation to reduce the amount of discarded drugs. And, of course, patients get little say in the matter, and it is they who may view the typical (noncapitated) approach as increasing their own costs needlessly, depending on their insurance coverage for the up to 20 percent not covered by Medicare Part B.

Rural hospitals, small clinics and physician's offices, and health care centers that serve underserved populations face additional challenges to reduce discarded drugs because of financial constraints. They may lack the appropriate resources to remove a portion of the vial contents for a given patient sterilely and return the unused portion to a refrigerator. According to a 2020 analysis, there are currently 1,844 rural community hospitals in the United States (Topchik et al., 2020). The analysis focused on the financial and operational data for 3 years before closure for closed hospitals and concluded that one in four rural hospitals are at risk of closure due to steady declines of operating margin and revenue (Topchik et al., 2020).

Even when the resources are available to keep the open vial following approved guidelines, in rural settings, it is unlikely that the vial would be fully used within the approved period, largely because the patient population is more dispersed. The sparseness of the population limits these providers' ability to share drugs among patients, as is done with batching.

Given the variety of incentives and barriers, depending on the organizational structure of the health care provider and the demographics of the patient population they serve, one single approach to reducing discarded drugs will likely not work for all providers.

KEY FINDINGS

1. *Recent legislation has been proposed to regulate payments for discarded drugs. Several of these bills proposed rebates from manufacturers directed to providers and payers for discarded drug amounts. Most bills did not propose rebates directed to patients, who would continue to be responsible for a portion of the cost of discarded drugs that were not used in their care.*

2. *Technological advances, such as closed-system drug transfer devices, show promise as potential ways to reduce the amount of discarded drugs with minimal or no risk to the patient.*

3. *To reduce the amount of discarded drug, clinical support staff may work to coordinate schedules so that patients requiring treatment of the same drug are scheduled within several hours of each other. This imposes logistical hurdles for practices and may create inconveniences for patients.*

CONCLUSIONS

1. Vial sharing and other clinical practices such as dose banding and dose rounding are possible mechanisms for reducing discarded drug. For small clinics and hospitals, vial sharing may be challenging to coordinate due to limited patient volume as well as the need to obtain special equipment to allow prolonged storage for safe drug use.

2. Several technologies and clinical strategies show promise for reducing discarded drugs from single-dose vials but are not encouraged by current policies or are not feasible without reducing current practice-based constraints.

3. Legislative initiatives proposing manufacturer rebates to providers and or payers for discarded drugs ignore the fact that a patient often would have been required to pay part of the cost of this discarded drug.

RECOMMENDATIONS[3]

RECOMMENDATION 4-1: The Secretary of the U.S. Department of Health and Human Services should direct the Centers for Medicare & Medicaid Services, the U.S. Food and Drug Administration, and the Centers for Disease Control and Prevention to initiate a partnership with other agencies, including the U.S. Department of Defense and the U.S. Department of Veterans Affairs, to work with health care and other organizations with expertise in areas such as industrial design and systems engineering to identify and implement technological systems that allow single-dose vials to be used safely across multiple patients.

RECOMMENDATION 4-2: The Secretary of the U.S. Department of Health and Human Services (HHS) should develop and implement policies that require drug manufacturers to produce injectable and infused drugs in multiple-dose vials when it is safe to do so. The Secretary of HHS should routinely review and evaluate the impact of such policies.

Because the committee's assessment shows that there is limited economic value to discarded drugs from single-dose vials under the current system in which drugs are developed, administered or paid for, a rebate strategy seems unlikely to achieve the intended goals. However, if the rebates that have been proposed in legislation are indeed implemented, the committee asserts that patients need to be included in those rebates.

RECOMMENDATION 4-3: In the event that legislation is enacted or regulatory action is taken to require rebates from manufacturers for discarded drugs, the U.S. Congress should require that rebates be directed first to cover the patient's out-of-pocket expense for the discarded drug and thereafter to health care providers and payers.

---

[3] These recommendations will be discussed fully in Chapter 6.

REFERENCES

Amerine, L. B., S. W. Savage, E. C. Rowe, R. Daniels, J. M. Valgus, R. Redding, and S. F. Eckel. 2019. Implementation of drug vial optimization to reduce drug waste. *Oncology Issues* 34(2):44–50.

ASCO (American Society of Clinical Oncology). 2018. *American Society of Clinical Oncology position statement: Pharmacy benefit managers and their impact on cancer care.* https://www.asco.org/sites/new-www.asco.org/files/content-files/advocacy-and-policy/documents/2018%20ASCO%20PBM%20Statement.pdf (accessed August 5, 2020).

ASHP (American Society of Health-System Pharmacists). 2019. *Drug products, labeling, and packaging.* https://www.ashp.org/-/media/assets/policy-guidelines/docs/policy-positions/policy-positions-drug-products-labeling-packaging.ashx (accessed August 5, 2020).

Becton, Dickinson and Company. 2020. *BD Phaseal™ system.* https://www.bd.com/en-us/offerings/capabilities/hazardous-drug-safety/phaseal-system (accessed August 5, 2020).

Chatelut, E., M. L. White-Koning, R. H. Mathijssen, F. Puisset, S. D. Baker, and A. Sparreboom. 2012. Dose banding as an alternative to body surface area-based dosing of chemotherapeutic agents. *British Journal of Cancer* 107(7):1100–1106.

De Prijck, K., E. D'Haese, J. Vandenbroucke, W. Coucke, H. Robays, and H. J. Nelis. 2008. Microbiological challenge of four protective devices for the reconstitution of cytotoxic agents. *Letters in Applied Microbiology* 47(6):543–548.

Dela Pena, J., K. Eschenburg, V. LaRocca, and D. Patel. 2020. *Financial impact of an automatic oncology drug rounding initiative: One year analysis.* Presented at HOPA 16th Annual Conference. March 11–14, Tampa, Florida.

Dobson, G., D. Tilson, and V. Tilson. 2015. Optimizing the timing and number of batches for compounded sterile products in an in-hospital pharmacy. *Decision Support Systems* 76(C):53–62.

Edwards, M. S., D. A. Solimando, F. R. Grollman, J. L. Pang, A. H. Chasick, C. M. Hightman, A. D. Johnson, M. G. Mickens, and L. M. Preston. 2013. Cost savings realized by use of the phaseal closed-system transfer device for preparation of antineoplastic agents. *Journal of Oncology Pharmacy Practice* 19(4):338–347.

Fahey, O. G., S. M. Koth, J. J. Bergsbaken, H. A. Jones, and P. J. Trapskin. 2020. Automated parenteral chemotherapy dose-banding to improve patient safety and decrease drug costs. *Journal of Oncology Pharmacy Practice* 26(2):345–350.

Fahrenbruch, R., P. Kintzel, A. M. Bott, S. Gilmore, and R. Markham. 2018. Dose rounding of biologic and cytotoxic anticancer agents: A position statement of the Hematology/Oncology Pharmacy Association. *Journal of Oncology Practice* 14(3):e130–e136.

Gilbar, P. J. 2020. Reducing cancer drug expenditure. *Presentation to the Committee on Implications of Discarded Weight-Based Drugs.* June 30.

Gilbar, P. J., and C. R. Chambers. 2018. How can we ensure value for money from expenditure on injectable cancer drugs? *Journal of Oncology Pharmacy Practice* 24(6):473–476.

Gilbar, P. J., C. R. Chambers, J. Vandenbrouche, P. J. Sessink, and T. G. Tyler. 2019. How can the use of closed system transfer devices to facilitate sharing of drug vials be optimised to achieve maximum cost savings? *Journal of Oncology Pharmacy Practice* 25(1):205–209.

Griggs, J. J., P. B. Mangu, H. Anderson, E. P. Balaban, J. J. Dignam, W. M. Hryniuk, V. A. Morrison, T. M. Pini, C. D. Runowicz, G. L. Rosner, M. Shayne, A. Sparreboom, L. E. Sucheston, and G. H. Lyman. 2012. Appropriate chemotherapy dosing for obese adult patients with cancer: American Society of Clinical Oncology clinical practice guideline. *Journal of Clinical Oncology* 30(13):1553–1561.

Guinto, J. B., and A. H. Szabatura. 2013. A perspective on dose banding. *Journal of the National Comprehensive Cancer Network* 11(3):357–359.

Hall, E., J. Zhang, E. J. Kim, G. Hwang, G. Chu, S. Bhatia, and S. Reddy. 2020. Economics of alternative dosing strategies for pembrolizumab and nivolumab at a single academic cancer center. *Cancer Medicine* 9(6):2106–2112.

HHS (U.S. Department of Health and Human Services). 2020. *HHS announces new public–private partnership to develop U.S.-based, high-speed emergency drug packaging solutions.* https://www.hhs.gov/about/news/2020/03/18/hhs-announces-new-public-private-partnership-to-develop-us-based-high-speed-emergency-drug-packaging-solutions.html (accessed September 4, 2020).

HOPA (Hematology/Oncology Pharmacy Association). 2019. *Intravenous cancer drug waste.* Issue Brief. http://www.hoparx.org/images/hopa/advocacy/Issue-Briefs/Drug_Waste_2019.pdf (accessed August 5, 2020).

Huertas, P., M. Cueto-Sola, P. Cava, C. García, A. Albert-Marí, E. Briz, and J. Andrés. 2015. Applying dose banding to the production of antineoplastic drugs: A narrative review of the literature. *Farmacia hospitalaria: Organo oficial de expresion cientifica de la Sociedad Espanola de Farmacia Hospitalaria* 39:210–216.

Johnson, K. B., C. K. K. Lee, S. A. Spooner, C. L. Davison, J. S. Helmke, and S. T. Weinberg. 2011. Automated dose-rounding recommendations for pediatric medications. *Pediatrics* 128(2):e422–e428.

Juhász, Á., G. Batka, and A. Szücs. 2016. Responding to drug shortages and rising costs: IV chemotherapy drug use optimization achieved by closed safety devices in hospital pharmacies. *Drugs & Therapy Perspectives* 32(4):170–176.

Lotvin, A. M., W. H. Shrank, S. C. Singh, B. P. Falit, and T. A. Brennan. 2014. Specialty medications: Traditional and novel tools can address rising spending on these costly drugs. *Health Affairs* 33(10):1736–1744.

Lyman, G. H. 2011. Commentary: Chemotherapy dosing in obese patients with cancer—the need for evidence-based clinical practice guidelines. *Journal of Oncology Practice* 7(1):17–18.

McMichael, D. M., D. M. Jefferson, E. T. Carey, R. A. Forrey, S. M. Spivey, J. M. Mulvaney, J. A. Jorgenson, and R. D. Haughs. 2011. Utility of the Phaseal closed system drug transfer device. *American Journal of Pharmacy Benefits* 3(1):9–16.

NIH (National Institutes of Health). 2020. *NIH to launch public–private partnership to speed COVID-19 vaccine and treatment options.* https://www.nih.gov/research-training/medical-research-initiatives/activ (accessed September 4, 2020).

Oswald, K. 2016. Chemotherapy dose banding to be rolled out across England. *The Pharmaceutical Journal* 296(7890).

Plumridge, R. J., and G. J. Sewell. 2001. Dose-banding of cytotoxic drugs: A new concept in cancer chemotherapy. *American Journal of Health-System Pharmacy* 58(18):1760–1764.

Politico. 2020. FDA says Pfizer vaccine vials hold extra doses, expanding supply. https://www.politico.com/news/2020/12/16/pfizer-vaccine-extra-doses-447117?cid=apn (accessed December 18, 2020).

Pouliquen, A. L., L. Escalup, N. Jourdan, P. Cottu, P. Faure, and I. Madelaine-Chambrin. 2011. Dose standardisation of anticancer drugs. *International Journal of Clinical Pharmacy* 33(2):221–228.

Rustemi, F., L. Malaj, E. Hoti, and E. Balla. 2019. Cost reduction as a result of bortezomib vial sharing in the University Hospital Center "Mother Theresa" Tirana. *European Journal of Hospital Pharmacy: Science and Practice* 26(4):239–240.

Simon, N., M. Vasseur, M. Pinturaud, M. Soichot, C. Richeval, L. Humbert, M. Lebecque, O. Sidikou, C. Barthelemy, and P. Bonnabry. 2016. Effectiveness of a closed-system transfer device in reducing surface contamination in a new antineoplastic drug-compounding unit: A prospective, controlled, parallel study. *PLOS ONE* 11(7):e0159052.

Smith, R. 2015. A 2-year retrospective review of vial sharing options for the compounding of cytotoxics. *European Journal of Hospital Pharmacy: Science and Practice* 22:161–164.

Spivey, S., and T. H. Connor. 2003. Determining sources of workplace contamination with antineoplastic drugs and comparing conventional IV drug preparation with a closed system. *Hospital Pharmacy* 38(2):135–139.

Suzuki, S., P. Gilbar, B. Yu, C. Matsuyama, and M. Yamaguchi. 2019. Current status of drug vial optimization use to prevent waste associated with injectable anticancer agents. *Journal of Oncology Pharmacy Practice* 25(1):244–246.

Topchik, M., K. Gross, M. Pinette, T. Brown, B. Balfour, and H. Kein. 2020. The rural health safety net under pressure: Rural hospital vulnerability. Chicago, IL: Chartis Center for Rural Health, The Chartis Group.

USP (United States Pharmacopeia). 2019. *USP compounding standards and beyond-use dates (buds).* https://www.usp.org/sites/default/files/usp/document/our-work/compounding/usp-bud-factsheet.pdf (accessed August 17, 2020).

Watanabe, J. H., D. L. Chau, and J. D. Hirsch. 2018. Federal and individual spending on the 10 costliest medications in Medicare Part D from 2011 to 2015. *Journal of the American Geriatrics Society* 66(8):1621–1624.

Wick, C., M. H. Slawson, J. A. Jorgenson, and L. S. Tyler. 2003. Using a closed-system protective device to reduce personnel exposure to antineoplastic agents. *American Journal of Health-System Pharmacy* 60(22):2314–2320.

5

Discarded Weight-Based Drugs in Single-Dose Vials

As discussed in the previous chapter, clinicians, health care systems, and others are trying to find more efficient and cost-effective ways to treat patients with weight-based drugs. These efforts have been prompted in large part by the high prices of these treatments, particularly in the United States but also in other countries. Given the large volume of weight-based, single-dose drugs discarded each year, a major challenge facing those interested in improving the efficiency of the system in which drugs are developed, administered or paid for, is determining how to calculate the value of that discarded drug. It is easy enough to multiply the per-milliliter cost of a drug by the number of milliliters discarded each year to get a putative value for the portion that is not administered (how much is discarded) and then add up all such drugs to get a total, but interpreting that number as the "value" of the discarded drugs is problematic. These typical calculations produce only nominal values that are based on the assumption that one can assign a value to an ounce of discarded drug that is equal to the value of an ounce of the drug in an unused vial. They do not accurately capture the economic value of discarded drugs and do not reflect the reality of the excess costs to patients and the system. This is because of the factors that go into determining the price of drugs in this country. In particular, it is not at all clear that a successful effort to reduce perceived drug *waste* would result in the sort of cost savings implied by such a simple calculation—or any cost savings at all. This chapter discusses how the issue of discarded drugs falls within the larger context of drug pricing, makes the economic case for why *waste* is not the right construct to analyze discarded drugs, offers a different way of thinking about the issue of *waste* in discarded weight-based drugs, draws the distinction between short-term and long-term approaches to address the issue, and suggests efficient ways to reduce the quantity of discarded drugs while ensuring patient safety.

WHY ARE DRUGS SO EXPENSIVE?

If the weight-based drugs in single-dose vials cost patients and payers only a few dollars—or even a few hundreds of dollars—routinely discarding significant amounts would not seem so serious. However, these vials are often thousands of dollars apiece, which makes discarding 20 or 30 percent of one seem wasteful. To calculate the value of this perceived waste from an economic perspective, it is critical to first understand how drugs are developed and prices are typically determined.

Drug Research and Development

The U.S. biopharmaceutical system is both extremely complex and opaque, and it can be difficult, if not impossible, to understand the reasons a particular drug is priced as it is. The most common explanation offered for the high price of drugs in the United States is the high cost of discovering a potential drug and bringing it to market. The cost of this process, which typically takes between 12 and 15 years, has been estimated to be between $757 million (Prasad and Mailankody, 2017) and $2.6 billion (DiMasi et al., 2016). Although there is no disagreement that the costs of drug discovery are large, there is widespread disagreement about exactly how large the costs of biopharmaceutical research and development are (NASEM, 2018).

To eventually show a profit, a biopharmaceutical company must make enough money on a drug's sales to cover the development, production, and marketing cost for the drug, as well as the costs related to developing drugs that never make it to market—and do it before the drug patent expires. After that, generic or biosimilar[1] manufacturers will typically begin to offer lower-priced versions and take a significant amount of sales away from the original developer. Prices typically fall by 20–30 percent with the first generic entrant and by 80 percent when several generics are in the market (Olson and Wendling, 2013). Introducing generics can lead to price competition, where the developer of the branded drug typically drops its

[1] A biosimilar is a biological drug that is very much like another biological drug (called the *reference drug*) that has already been approved by the U.S. Food and Drug Administration. Biosimilar drugs and reference drugs are made from living organisms but may be made in different ways and of slightly different substances.

price significantly to compete with the generic versions, but prices may not decline as rapidly with specialty drugs (Cole and Dusetzina, 2018).

While the high cost of developing drugs may be offered as a justification for high drug prices and certainly imply that biopharmaceutical companies would not keep developing new drugs if they did not expect to be paid well for their efforts, the research and development costs actually explain only a part of the high costs of drugs in the United States.

Patent Protections

Basic patent protection for a new drug lasts for 20 years from the date the application is filed, which generally takes place soon after a potential use for a drug is discovered. Since the development, testing, and approval process can take a decade or more, a drug company can be left with a relatively few years of patent protection once a drug goes to market. The Hatch-Waxman Act of 1984[2] addressed this by making it possible to extend the effective patent life. Drug companies also use a variety of legal maneuvers to extend their period of exclusivity beyond that basic period, a strategy known as "evergreening" (Dwivedi et al., 2010; NASEM, 2018). The goal of patent protection is to make sure that drug developers have the chance to profit before facing competition from others that did not have the risk and expense of developing and testing the new drug. However, some have charged that the system works too well, and there is some evidence for this, as drug companies as a group consistently have higher profit margins than companies in almost any other sector (Chen, 2015; Sood et al., 2017).

Production Cost

One factor that does not play a particularly large role in the prices of new infused or injectable drugs is the manufacturing cost. Compared with research and development costs, manufacturing is relatively cheap—which is why generic drugs and biosimilars can be sold at such low prices compared to new, patent-protected drugs. In fact, the most profitable way for a patent-holding drug manufacturer to price drugs would be to set that price based on a payer's willingness to pay for a course of treatment and then ship the drug in packages of whatever size were most economical (Glied and Sampat, 2016). The manufacturing itself does not drive the price.

---

[2] Drug Price Competition and Patent Term Restoration Act of 1984, Public Law 98-417, 98th Congress (September 24, 1984).

Perceived Value and Willingness to Pay

On the demand side, an equally important factor in drug pricing is the payer's willingness to pay. Drugs that are difficult and therefore costly to produce would not command high prices if consumers had no demand for them. Payers include the individual receiving the drug (or family members), the individual's health insurance plan, and governmental programs, such as Medicare or Medicaid. This willingness to pay depends in turn on the drug's value or perceived value. A drug that is more effective against a serious disease or increases survival rates more than existing alternatives can be priced higher than its competitors, and the larger the improvement, the higher the possible price. However, many new drugs with relatively modest advantages over existing drugs are still priced significantly higher (Frank et al., 2020; Vokinger et al., 2020).

Current reimbursement approaches, incentives for intermediaries in the drug supply chain, and insurance design are also important elements affecting observed willingness to pay. Medicare is constrained by its inability to exclude drugs from coverage, which means that Medicare cannot refuse to cover drugs that are significantly more costly than alternatives with similar performance (see, e.g., NASEM, 2018). Under the current approach of paying for clinician-administered drugs, health care providers are paid based on the drug's prices. Simultaneously, intermediaries, such as pharmacy benefit managers (PBMs), manage drug formularies to define the lists of drugs that a health care provider can administer to a patient and receive reimbursement for based on the individual's health insurance plan. Therefore, in addition to the payers, health care providers, who often choose which drugs to use, also need to be convinced of the benefit of new drugs.

In brief, U.S. drug prices are the product of a complex and confusing system, one in which many of the components are hidden from outside observers. While the main forces at work are clear—the high cost of research and development, patent protections, new drugs' real or perceived value, and the willingness of payers, including health insurers and patients, to pay—how these factors and others interact to determine the price of a particular drug is far from clear.

APPROACHES TO MANAGING DRUG COSTS

The United States pays more for prescription drugs than any other industrialized country (Kanavos et al., 2013; Sarnak et al., 2017). In 2018, the Assistant Secretary for Planning and Evaluation conducted a study that compared the prices that Medicare paid for selected Part B drugs with the prices paid in 16 other industrialized countries (ASPE, 2020) and concluded that prices in the United States were 1.8 times higher. A previous

National Academies of Sciences, Engineering, and Medicine (National Academies) report, *Making Medicines Affordable: A National Imperative*, proposed a range of approaches to help prevent drug expenditures from spiraling out of control. A brief overview of those approaches for managing the availability and affordability of prescription drugs for all Americans is discussed next. In the United States the cost of drugs to patients is ultimately the result of negotiations among health insurance companies, drug companies, and intermediaries (such as PBMs) and the type of health insurance coverage and benefit design.

Insights from the *Making Medicines Affordable* Report

Making Medicines Affordable (NASEM, 2018) examined in detail the factors influencing prescription drug prices in the United States and offered a list of suggested actions for reducing drug costs. Briefly, the report concluded that the high cost of prescription drugs is likely due to a combination of factors—not just the expense of discovering and developing the drugs—although the complexity of the U.S. health care system makes it difficult to know exactly how large a role any given factor plays. In the United States the cost of drugs to patients is ultimately the result of negotiations among health insurance companies, drug companies, and intermediaries (such as PBMs) and the type of health insurance coverage and benefit design. Different patients can pay vastly different amounts for the same drug depending on their health benefit design. Various factors influence these negotiations, including the costs of developing and marketing drugs, the benefits of a drug, and how it compares with other drugs and treatments.

The report detailed several specific factors beyond the costs of developing and marketing. For example, large health insurance companies influence the cost of drugs by deciding whether they will cover the cost for each drug in a given situation and how much cost-sharing the patient will be responsible for. Intermediaries, such as PBMs, have their own influence too. They act as agents for insurance companies and large employers to negotiate drug prices with manufacturers and retail pharmacies and manage formularies on behalf of payers. These factors and many others interact in complex and often nontransparent ways to influence drug costs, and it is not at all clear how to go about lowering drug prices in the United States without unintended consequences, such as potentially slowing down the drug development pipeline (NASEM, 2018).

In light of the various factors driving the high drug costs, the report offered eight specific recommendations, each with associated implementation actions, to improve the affordability of prescription drugs without discouraging continued innovation in drug development:

- Accelerate the market entry and use of generics and biosimilars.
- Consolidate governmental purchasing power, strengthen formulary design, and improve drug valuation methods.
- Ensure greater transparency of financial flows and profit margins in the biopharmaceutical supply chain.
- Discourage direct-to-consumer advertising of prescription drugs.
- Design insurance benefits to mitigate patient drug cost burdens.
- Improve federal discount programs to aid vulnerable populations.
- Ensure financial incentives for rare diseases are not extended to widely sold drugs.
- Implement reimbursement incentives that align with value.

Box 5-1 highlights some of the implementation actions from the report that relate directly to the Medicare program and its beneficiaries.

BOX 5-1
Select Implementation Actions from the 2018 National Academies Report *Making Medicines Affordable: A National Imperative*

Recommendation B-1: The U.S. Congress should modify existing legislation so as to allow the U.S. Department of Health and Human Services, acting as a single entity, to directly negotiate prices with producers and suppliers of medicines, including acting on behalf of any relevant state agency that elects to participate in the process.

Recommendation B-3: The U.S. Congress should authorize the U.S. Department of Health and Human Services, related federal agencies, and associated private payers to expand flexibility in formulary design, including the selective exclusion of drugs in certain cases, such as when less costly drugs provide a similar clinical benefit.

Recommendation E-1: The U.S. Congress should establish limits on the total annual out-of-pocket costs paid by enrollees in Medicare Part D plans that cover prescription drugs by removing the cost-sharing requirement for patients who reach the catastrophic coverage limit.

Recommendation E-2: The U.S. Congress should direct the Centers for Medicare & Medicaid Services to modify the designs of plans offered through Medicare Part D and governmental health insurance exchanges to limit patients' out-of-pocket payments for drugs when there is clear evidence that treatment adherence

Recommendation B-1—allowing the Secretary of the U.S. Department of Health and Human Services (HHS) to negotiate directly for drugs—relates to the topic of discarded drugs as follows: Medicare is the single largest purchaser of drugs in the United States, and Part B drugs are among the most expensive drugs. In the United States, drug manufacturers set their own prices and can simply adjust their prices to maintain their revenues in response to efforts to lower the expense of using drugs (discussed in more detail later in this chapter). The current reimbursement system for most Part B drugs is based on the drug's ASP plus a percentage add-on. The dollar amount of the add-on for a drug is larger when the drug price is high, thereby increasing patients' cost-sharing responsibility and raising spending on Part B drugs for Medicare and patients.

According to a survey by the Kaiser Family Foundation, nearly 90 percent of the public favors allowing the federal government to negotiate

for a particular indication can reduce the total cost of care, as determined by the U.S. Department of Health and Human Services.

Recommendation E-3: The U.S. Congress should direct the Centers for Medicare & Medicaid Services to specify that when patient cost-sharing is calculated as a fraction of drug prices in insurance policies through Medicare Part D and governmental health insurance exchanges, this calculation should be based on net prices, not list prices. All state and private prescription drug plans should be encouraged to follow this approach.

Recommendation E-4: The U.S. Congress should require the Centers for Medicare & Medicaid Services, when determining patient cost-sharing rates, to specifically include the costs and the clinical effectiveness of prescription drugs and available treatment alternatives. This evaluation should address, where feasible, the total costs of care rather than simply the costs of the drugs themselves.

Recommendation H-1: Payers should establish payment policies for drugs administered by clinicians in medical practices and hospitals that do not differentiate for the site of care (site neutral payment).

Recommendation H-3: Payers should eliminate the practice of reimbursing clinicians and stand-alone and hospital-based clinics on the basis of list prices for drugs covered under the Medicare medical benefit, and replace the current reimbursement model with fixed fees that support clinical care and the costs of storing and administering these drugs.

SOURCE: NASEM, 2018.

drug prices for Medicare (Cubanski et al., 2019). Several lawmakers have introduced bills to change the law and allow government drug price negotiation. (Box 5-2 presents a summary of some of the recent bills related to drug negotiation.) While the bills seek to achieve the same overall goal of price negotiation, they take different approaches. Currently, Medicare has very limited authority to exclude drugs from its formulary. Enabling HHS to negotiate drug prices for all Medicare enrollees would increase its bargaining power with drug manufacturers. Furthermore, giving it the authority to negotiate drug prices would provide the leverage needed to lower drug costs, particularly for high-priced drugs that have no competitors.

ECONOMICS OF PACKAGING WEIGHT-BASED DRUGS

For weight-based drugs, two patients with the same condition and the same severity who are prescribed the same drug will generally receive different amounts of that drug. This leads to a fundamental question

BOX 5-2
Select Draft Bills Related to Drug Negotiation

S. 62, Empowering Medicare Seniors to Negotiate Drug Prices Act of 2019: This would allow the Centers for Medicare & Medicaid Services (CMS) to negotiate drug prices under the Medicare prescription drug benefit and institute a price structure for the reimbursement of drugs covered under Medicare.

S. 377 and H.R. 1046, Medicare Negotiation and Competitive Licensing Act of 2019: This would require CMS to negotiate with pharmaceutical companies regarding prices for drugs covered under the Medicare prescription drug benefit. The bill notes that CMS must consider certain factors, including the clinical effectiveness and cost-effectiveness of the drug, the financial burden on patients, and unmet patient needs during negotiations.

S. 99 and H.R. 448, Medicare Drug Price Negotiation Act: This would require CMS to negotiate the prices of covered drugs and either establish a formulary for covered drugs or require changes to prescription drug plan formularies that take into account CMS negotiations.

H.R. 3, Elijah E. Cummings Lower Drug Costs Now Act of 2019: This would require the Secretary of the U.S. Department of Health and Human Services to negotiate the price of brand-name drugs without generic competitors and would make the negotiated price available to both Medicare and private payers. The bill would also require pharmaceutical manufacturers to pay rebates to Medicare if the price of their drugs increased faster than inflation.

concerning the distribution of such drugs: given that the drug cannot always be packaged into one-size-fits-all doses that will be dispensed to everyone who needs them, how should they be packaged?

One approach would be to sell the drugs in larger amounts that could be divided among multiple patients. If, for example, a drug in liquid form was provided in 25-mL containers, Patient A might get a 3.5-mL dose, Patient B a 6-mL dose, Patient C a 4-mL dose, and so on until the container was used up and a new one was opened. This approach has various problems, both medical and practical, however. A major concern is that once the seal on the drug container has been broken, contamination from various sources—not just other patients but the many hazards that can be found in a hospital or a doctor's office—becomes an issue. Additionally, once opened, the drug has a limited lifetime, during which it must all be used, or else the remainder will be discarded.

These considerations led to the current system in which weight-based drugs are packaged in smaller quantities that are intended for a single use, but this creates another set of issues centered on the basic question of how to determine the best sizes for these packages. Drug companies begin thinking about this issue at the clinical trial stage, when they are also considering the dose strength and volume. This is true for approval for the first indication but not for subsequent indications. Once the dose strength and volume have been determined, the quantity of the drug that a given patient will need is easily calculated.

How big should the vials be? In the example given above, a single 6-mL vial (plus a certain amount of required overfill) would be enough for all adults up to 100 kg, but half the vial would have to be discarded with a 50-kg patient. Or the drug could be distributed in both 3-mL and 6-mL sizes, which would sharply decrease the amount of unused drug for people who weigh 50 kg or less but would make no difference for anyone between 50 and 100 kg. Offering the drug in three vial sizes—3 mL, 4.5 mL, 6 mL—would do even more to decrease the amounts of drugs discarded in various situations.

However, increasing the number of vial sizes comes at a cost. The development of each vial size will require the manufacturing process to be validated, and its labeling and shipping systems will also need to be developed and validated. In some cases, new parts or equipment would be required for the new production. The paperwork for each vial size must be filed in multiple countries, and each requires an inventory system and a global supply chain. This alternative would add complexity to manufacturing, transportation, and supply chain management. Thus, each additional vial size that is offered raises the overall cost of providing the drug, and drug companies look to balance the cost of the discarded drug versus the cost of offering multiple vial sizes.

VALUE OF UNUSED SINGLE-DOSE VIAL DRUGS

The discarded portions of single-dose vials are typically viewed as "wasted." After all, they were manufactured and distributed and, most often, paid for, but they were never used to treat patients, which would seem to be the very definition of *waste*. Simply adding up the discarded portions and valuing them on a simple per-milliliter basis leads to the conclusion that the U.S. health care system is discarding billions of dollars of weight-based drugs each year. But this interpretation does not capture the full picture of the value of these discarded drugs.

To understand why these discarded portions may not actually represent waste in an economic sense, the easiest place to start is with the standard calculation that people make when assigning a dollar value to this perceived waste: suppose a single-dose vial costs $2,000, and only 75 percent of that is used. Because one-quarter of $2,000 is $500, the conclusion is that $500 of the drug was wasted. This type of calculation underlies the various estimates that have been reported for the total dollar value of weight-based drugs that are "wasted" each year as explained in Chapter 3.

Hidden in this argument is a basic assumption—that every milligram of the drug in that vial has equal value and that, in particular, the unused milligrams are equal in value per milligram to the used milligrams. However, this is not how drugs are priced. The price of a drug is typically based not on how much is used but on the willingness to pay for the drug's therapeutic benefit. Put differently, because manufacturing costs do not drive drug prices, the quantity of a drug that a patient receives also does not drive pricing. In general, a patient cares only about getting a correct dose of the drug for a treatment. Thus, the patient—mostly likely through an insurance company or Medicare—has paid $2,000 for this dose and does not care how it was packaged. If the patient needs, say, 600 mg of a drug, the patient does not care if the vial holds 600 mg, 800 mg, or 1,200 mg or if it takes two vials with 400 mg each or any other combination. To the patient, the 600-mg dose is worth $2,000, and the remainder has no value whatsoever. Box 5-3 illustrates other ways to think about the concept of pricing according to what people are willing to pay.

ROLE OF REIMBURSEMENT IN SHAPING ATTITUDES TOWARD DISCARDED DRUGS

Pulling back to look at the issue of discarded drugs from single-dose vials in a broader context, it becomes clear that much of the concern about these discarded drugs has its roots in the particular approach to paying—and reimbursing health care providers—for them. Specifically,

BOX 5-3
Pricing According to What People Are Willing to Pay

For products that do not compete aggressively with another product through price, price is determined not by the cost of production but rather by individuals' willingness to pay for the product. For example, consider an individual who wants to bake a cake who bought a gallon of buttermilk for $2.80 but only ended up using about one quart and discarded the rest. By the above logic, the individual wasted $2.10 of the buttermilk, but that would only make sense if the unused buttermilk could be resold for $2.10. To this individual, the $2.80 was the cost of having buttermilk for the cake; the baker could choose to pay it or not, but either way, the unused amount was not part of the calculation. Furthermore, the individual probably could have bought just one quart of buttermilk—if he or she was willing to take the chance that this would be enough for the cake—but the price of that quart would not have been close to one-quarter of $2.80, or 70 cents. In reality, the cost of one quart of buttermilk in a grocery store is much closer to the $2.80 cost for a gallon than it is to 70 cents.[a]

A second way of thinking about the value of a weight-based drug or a container of buttermilk—the value placed on it by the seller rather than the consumer. Many things go into the cost of a container of buttermilk sitting on a shelf in a grocery store—not just production, but packaging, distributing, advertising, putting it on the shelf, and so on—which is why a gallon of buttermilk does not cost four times as much as one quart. This effect is even more pronounced with pharmaceuticals because almost all drugs have a relatively high fixed production cost and a relatively low marginal production cost. The fixed cost includes developing the drug and getting it approved, building a manufacturing plant, and creating the associated packaging and marketing materials. The marginal costs are important because the price that a manufacturer charges for a drug depends mainly on two things: marginal costs and willingness to pay for the treatment. And because the marginal costs are low, the price of drugs in the United States is determined mainly by willingness to pay.

As another example, consider an expensive item of clothing, such as a $3,000 coat. If two people, one very small and one very large, go into a store to purchase that coat, they will each pay the same $3,000 despite the fact that the XXL coat required much more material to construct. That is because the cost of the material is a very small part of the overall cost and the coat is worth no more to the very large person than to the very small person. When materials make up a negligible part of the overall cost, the manufacturer tends to set the price according to what people are willing to pay rather than according to what the item cost to make. This is true for products that do not face intensive competition (i.e., do not compete aggressively with another through price), since in these settings, price is determined not by the cost of production but rather by willingness to pay.

Or, to offer an example a bit closer in its details to single-dose vials, consider a $2,000 dress that needs to be altered to fit properly. Depending on the alteration, quite a bit of material might have to be cut off and discarded, but the customer does not typically get a rebate because all the fabric was not needed.

continued

BOX 5-3 Continued

The key message here is that in markets like the biopharmaceutical market, where the cost of production is just a fraction of the total product price, the marginal costs—the per-unit costs to produce or to buy additional product—are trivial and have very little relationship to the total cost. In particular, just as it would be a mistake to assume that the fabric discarded in an alteration is worth some fraction of the cost of the dress, it is a mistake to look at the per-unit cost of a drug and assume you can use that figure to place a value on the portion of drugs that are discarded from a single-use vial.

---

[a] Adapted from Dr. Amitabh Chandra's presentation to the committee at a public session.

the pricing and reimbursement for these drugs on a per-milliliter basis, with the cost for a particular treatment dependent on how much is used on that patient, carries with it the implication that each milliliter in a vial has its own inherent value equal to every other milliliter.

But this is not the only logical way to think about the discarded drugs. Consider, for example, a payment and reimbursement system in which every patient, no matter how much of the drug a treatment requires, pays exactly the same amount for it. This is how drugs are priced in many other countries (Roy, 2019). Furthermore, this is a typical approach to pricing in many other areas of the economy. As noted in Box 5-3, items of clothing, for instance, generally cost the same for all sizes, from XS to XXL, even though the largest sizes may need two or more times as much cloth as the smallest ones (and even if the fabric is relatively expensive).

Now suppose that this system were in place in the United States. How would that change the thinking about discarded drugs? In this situation, each patient would pay the same amount for a given treatment no matter how much of the drug was required—and the drug company would receive exactly the same amount for each patient, just like a clothing company selling coats. With a per-treatment cost, there would no longer be an implication that a percentage of a vial's value is wasted each time less than 100 percent of it is used. Specifically, in contrast with per-milliliter pricing, where there is an advantage to using the unused portion of a vial on a second patient as a way of saving money, per-treatment pricing suggests no such advantage. In theory, a health care provider could share vials, but there would be no reason to because there would be no savings—the money paid to the drug company would rely only on the number of patients treated, not on how much of the drug was used. With that approach to pricing, there would no longer be any need to calculate the amount of weight-based drugs that are discarded each year. Nothing important about the system would have changed—patients would still be getting the same treatments, and drug companies would still be getting paid about the same total amount, although some patients would be paying less and some more in a more equitable system—but the concerns about billions of dollars wasted each year on discarded drugs would vanish along with the additional administrative work needed to calculate how much drug was not administered.

Thus, any consideration of the issue of discarded weight-based drugs must take place in the larger context of how those drugs are priced and paid for.

LIKELY UNINTENDED CONSEQUENCES OF EFFORTS TO REDUCE DISCARDED DRUGS

At the committee's public sessions, several speakers discussed that many people believe that reducing the amount of discarded drugs from single-dose vials is unlikely to result in financial savings for patients because the prices of drugs are determined on the basis of willingness to pay for a treatment's outcome and not the specific amount of drug dispensed. Some observers believe that if clinicians, hospitals, and health systems are successful in reducing discarded drugs from single-dose vials or if payers (private or federal) promulgate policies to pay for volume dispensed, those efforts will eventually trigger drug companies to raise prices to compensate for their lost revenue. Ultimately, the per-patient price will reflect the average willingness of patients to pay, and the price of dosing units (e.g., a large vial of a drug) will reflect the number of patients each dosing unit can treat.

For example, suppose that patients—or Medicare, or insurance companies—are willing to pay $5,000 for a drug that comes in 5-mg vials ($1,000 per milligram), but the average patient needs only 3 mg. Now, suppose that through vial sharing or some other clinical practices discussed in Chapter 4, clinicians are able to treat three patients with two vials, so now they are paying $10,000 but for three patients instead of two. Basic economic theory would predict that drug companies are not going to keep the same pricing because they know that payers and patients are willing to pay $5,000 per treatment, so they increase the price to $7,500 per vial; now two vials cost $15,000, and it is back to $5,000 per treatment for three patients. However, in the real world, drug prices depend on multiple factors, including payers' negotiating power and public policies. Vial sharing or some other clinical practices to reduce discarded drugs could be more worthwhile under a scenario in which the government had a mechanism to negotiate prices or to limit increases in drug prices while acknowledging the need for reasonable profit margins for drug manufacturers. But this scenario does not currently apply in the United States.

This is the basic economic challenge with efforts to save money by cutting back on the perceived *waste* or designing payment policies that are focusing on reimbursing manufacturers per volume unit of drug dispensed. In the beginning, as long as only a few clinicians are able to reduce discarded drugs through vial sharing or some other clinical practice and that does not affect drug company revenue, the drug companies may be comfortable with it, but if the practice ever becomes widespread, including federal policy or policy by large health care payers, the drug companies would likely respond. The response does not have to be as simple as increasing the price but could involve changing the vial sizes, for instance—and the end result would be that the drug companies still derive the same revenue, but health care providers are doing a lot of extra work to treat multiple patients with a single vial, and the average consumer would pay about the same amount for a course of treatment. But it is not clear whether those price increases would wipe out all the savings achieved by the more efficient use of the drugs. Perhaps there would be some relatively small cost savings, or perhaps that savings would be overwhelmed by the costs of "saving" the discarded drugs, and the total cost to the system in which drugs are developed, administered, or paid for might be greater. Without a detailed economic analysis, it is impossible to predict.

KEY FINDINGS

1. *Differing perspectives about the definition of "drug waste" can lead to differing approaches to address the complexities that contribute to failure to administer all of the drug delivered in vials.*

2. *In the United States, agreement is lacking among stakeholders about whether requiring manufacturers to produce more vial sizes would result in any cost savings to the Medicare program and its beneficiaries.*

3. *The reimbursement of branded or patent-protected weight-based dose drugs is multifactorial and is more reflective of willingness to pay than the cost of production or development costs.*

CONCLUSIONS

1. Under the current system in which drugs are developed, administered, or paid for, when the drug is discarded, there is no money to recoup. Therefore, there is limited economic value to discarded injectable or infused drugs from single-dose vials.

2. Concerns about reducing discarded drug take place in the larger context of concerns about drug costs, and particularly the cost to patients, in the United States.

3. Under the current system in which drugs are developed, administered, or paid for, approaches to reduce the discarding of drugs from single-dose vials could have unintended consequences. Successful efforts may eventually trigger drug companies to raise the prices to derive constant or increased revenue for their products. Approaches to reducing discarded drugs from single-dose vials would need to leverage other strategies aimed at lowering drug prices, including allowing the Secretary of the U.S. Department of Health and Human Services to negotiate directly with manufacturers regarding the price of drugs.

RECOMMENDATION[3]

RECOMMENDATION 5-1: Drug developers, health care providers, and payers should focus their efforts on reducing inefficiencies in drug development, delivery, and payment systems that lead to excess costs for both the health care system and for patients rather than on trying to recoup payments associated with the discarded drugs.

REFERENCES

ASPE (Office of the Assistant Secretary for Planning and Evaluation). 2020. *Medicare Part B spending*. https://aspe.hhs.gov/medicare-part-b (accessed August 7, 2020).

Chen, L. 2015. *The most profitable industries in 2016*. https://www.forbes.com/sites/liyanchen/2015/12/21/the-most-profitable-industries-in-2016/#284d4e7b5716 (accessed August 7, 2020).

Cole, A. L., and S. B. Dusetzina. 2018. Generic price competition for specialty drugs: Too little, too late?. *Health Affairs* 37(5):738–742.

Cubanski, J., T. Neuman, S. True, and M. Freed. 2019. *What's the latest on Medicare drug price negotiations?* KFF Issue Brief. http://files.kff.org/attachment/Issue-Brief-Whats-the-Latest-on-Medicare-Drug-Price-Negotiations (accessed August 31, 2020).

[3] This recommendation will be discussed fully in Chapter 6.

DiMasi, J. A., H. G. Grabowski, and R. W. Hansen. 2016. Innovation in the pharmaceutical industry: New estimates of R&D costs. *Journal of Health Economics* 47:20–33.

Dwivedi, G., S. Hallihosur, and L. Rangan. 2010. Evergreening: A deceptive device in patent rights. *Technology in Society* 32(4):324–330.

Frank, R. G., J. Avorn, and A. S. Kesselheim. 2020. What do high drug prices buy us? *Health Affairs Blog*. April 29, 2020. doi: 10.1377/hblog20200424.131397.

Glied, S., and B. Sampat. 2016. *Would a wider variety of vial sizes reduce the cost of chemotherapy? Not likely*. https://www.healthaffairs.org/do/10.1377/hblog20160511.054821/full (accessed December 9, 2020).

Kanavos, P., A. Ferrario, S. Vandoros, and G. F. Anderson. 2013. Higher U.S. branded drug prices and spending compared to other countries may stem partly from quick uptake of new drugs. *Health Affairs* 32(4):753–761.

NASEM (National Academies of Sciences, Engineering, and Medicine). 2018. *Making medicines affordable: A national imperative*. Washington, DC: The National Academies Press.

Olson, L., and B. W. Wendling. 2013. *The effect of generic drug competition on generic drug prices during the Hatch–Waxman 180-day exclusivity period*. Working Paper No. 317. Washington, DC: Federal Trade Commission Bureau of Economics. https://www.ftc.gov/sites/default/files/documents/reports/estimating-effect-entry-generic-drug-prices-using-hatch-waxman-exclusivity/wp317.pdf (accessed October 29, 2020)

Prasad, V., and S. Mailankody. 2017. Research and development spending to bring a single cancer drug to market and revenues after approval. *JAMA Internal Medicine* 177(11):1569–1575.

Roy, A. 2019. *What Medicare can learn from other countries on drug pricing*. Foundation for Research on Equal Opportunity. https://freopp.org/what-medicare-can-learn-from-other-countries-on-drug-pricing-bf298d390bc5 (accessed April 29, 2020).

Sarnak, D. O., D. Squires, G. Kuzmak, and S. Bishop. 2017. Paying for prescription drugs around the world: Why is the U.S. an outlier? *Commonwealth Fund Issue Brief* 1–14.

Sood, N., K. Van Nuys. T. Shih, and D. Goldman. 2017. Follow the money: The flow of funds in the pharmaceutical distribution system. *Health Affairs Blog*. June 13. doi: 10.1377/hblog20170613.060557.

Vokinger, K. N., T. J. Hwang, T. Grischott, S. Reichert, A. Tibau, T. Rosemann, and A. S. Kesselheim. 2020. Prices and clinical benefit of cancer drugs in the USA and Europe: A cost–benefit analysis. *The Lancet Oncology* 21(5):664–670.

6

Prescription for Reducing Discarded Drugs

The study committee was charged with examining the federal health care costs, safety, and quality concerns associated with discarded drugs that result from weight-based dosing of medicines contained in single-dose vials. In this chapter, the committee summarizes its goals and recommendations for policy, practice, and research as they relate to the study's charge.

Understanding the ways in which drug *waste* is conceptualized is an important part of any approach to address the costs associated with discarded excess drugs contained in single-dose vials. As discussed in previous chapters, on the surface it can seem extremely wasteful that health care providers discard significant portions of the drug in single-dose vials that can cost thousands of dollars. And, indeed, it is that appearance of significant waste that has led observers to attempt to calculate the total value of drugs "wasted" in this way each year and to look for ways to minimize this *waste*. However, as discussed in Chapter 5, the concept of *waste* is not the appropriate construct for assessing and addressing the issue of discarded drugs. Rather, the primary focus should be on the marginal costs of producing the drugs and the factors that go into determining their pricing and paying for them.

Any decision made by U.S. policy makers or regulators would have global implications because the United States is the biggest worldwide purchaser of drugs, and regulators in the rest of the world often follow U.S. Food and Drug Administration (FDA) guidance. Therefore, appropriate conceptualization of discarded drugs is vital for policy makers to understand the trade-offs among different approaches for addressing the problem.

The fundamental issues addressed by this report can inform an overarching approach to understanding the causes and implications of the large amount of discarded drugs and to reducing certain inefficiencies in the system in which drugs are developed, administered, or paid for. This could set a precedent that the rest of the world may choose to adopt.

GOALS AND RECOMMENDATIONS

The committee's analysis of the economics of weight-based drugs in single-dose vials (see Chapter 5) led them to a single profound conclusion:

> ***Under the current system in which drugs are developed, administered, or paid for, when the drug is discarded, there is no money to recoup. Therefore, there is limited economic value to discarded injectable or infused drugs from single-dose vials.***

While the committee asserts there is little recoverable value to discarded drugs, it does see several opportunities to reduce inefficiencies that could lead to cost savings and improve the quality of care for patients. Therefore, the committee's overarching recommendation[1] is:

> **RECOMMENDATION 5-1: Drug developers, health care providers, and payers should focus their efforts on reducing inefficiencies in drug development, delivery, and payment systems that lead to excess costs for both the health care system and for patients rather than on trying to recoup payments associated with the discarded drugs.**

To lay the foundation for strategies to reduce certain inefficiencies that lead to discarded drugs while ensuring patient safety and quality care, the committee presents **two broad goals** and **eight associated recommendations.** The goals and proposed actions are oriented toward changing incentives and increasing efficiency in how these drugs are developed, administered, and paid for. The committee recognizes that successfully addressing the issue of discarded drugs will necessitate an implementation process that requires effective collaborations and efforts by all stakeholders in the biopharmaceutical supply chain. Therefore, in formulating its recommendations, the committee has considered the ways in which a proposed action could change if another is not carried out. In this sense,

---

[1] The committee's recommendations are numbered according to the chapter of the main report in which they first appear. Thus, Recommendation 5-1 is in Chapter 5.

the committee's recommendations should ideally be viewed as a "package." The committee's recommendations, restated below, are supported by the findings and conclusions at the end of previous chapters.

Goal 1: Promote the Effective, Efficient, and Safe Use of Infused or Injectable Drugs

Weight-based dosing (which, for the purposes of this report, includes dosing based on body surface area [BSA]) is a common method for dose determination for infused and injectable drugs because of how early drug testing and clinical trials are currently conducted. The dosing for a drug is determined in the clinical trials that are performed, typically during the early stages of the development process, to demonstrate that the drug is safe and effective. As discussed in Chapter 2, the dosing that is ultimately shown to be safe and effective in pivotal trials is the one that regulators will approve for marketing. Pivotal trials are intended to provide the evidence and data that FDA ultimately uses to decide whether to approve a potential new medicine. Thus, if weight-based dosing is used in these pivotal trials, then a weight-based dosing regimen will be approved. Evidence from other dosing practices, such as dose banding and dose capping, suggests that alternatives to weight-based dosing might be just as safe and effective for many indications, but pivotal trials rarely compare weight-based dosing with other methods.

Empirical evidence supporting the use of weight-based dosing instead of fixed dosing for injectable or infused drugs is limited.

The use of trials considering different dosing strategies (e.g., weight based versus fixed dose) early in the drug development process could help to determine if dosing based on a patient's body size (e.g., weight or body surface area) provides greater benefit than a fixed dose for a given therapeutic agent.

RECOMMENDATION 2-1: The U.S. Food and Drug Administration should require sponsors of pivotal trials for new or extended therapeutic indications to use fixed dosing for a given clinical indication unless safety and efficacy would be compromised. Manufacturers of products already in the market should consider conducting additional studies after approval so that these drugs can, when indicated, be converted to fixed dosing.

Drugs contained in a single-dose vial are intended to be used a single time for a single patient. Single-dose vials usually do not contain antimicrobial preservatives that help prevent contamination from bacterial growth, which is why the remainder is typically discarded immediately after a dose is drawn. Multiple-dose vials, however, are intended to contain more than one dose. They have preservatives to stop bacterial growth but can be contaminated if safe injection practices are not followed. To complicate matters, current federal policies, research, and practice relevant to the costs associated with discarded drugs contained in single-dose vials are fragmented across a variety of agencies and professional organizations.

The committee has identified significant conflicts among the safety concerns that motivate the regulatory guidance on the repackaging of single-dose drugs—that is, dividing the content of a single-dose vial into multiple individual doses—by pertinent federal agencies. For example, according to FDA, using multiple single-dose vials to treat a single patient can lead to medication errors and sharing a single vial among multiple patients can lead to contamination. However, the Centers for Medicare & Medicaid Services (CMS) permits health care providers to administer repackaged doses to multiple patients, provided that each repackaged dose is used for a single patient. In contrast, guidance from the Centers for Disease Control and Prevention (CDC) states that vials labeled by the manufacturer as single dose or single use should be used only for one patient and repackaging is not acceptable.

A number of other Organisation for Economic Co-operation and Development (OECD) countries have well-established clinical and operational approaches that allow for delivering medication to multiple patients from a single vial through vial sharing. Several others have promoted the use of standardized doses. For example, dose banding, a clinical practice in which drug doses that fall within predefined ranges established through clinical calculations are rounded up or down for patients, is widely used in the United Kingdom and other parts of Europe. Such upward or downward rounding is typically designed to allow use of a complete vial, without discarding any medication.

Nonetheless, efforts to standardize the delivery of medication to multiple patients from a single-dose vial, when necessary and allowed, currently entail practical operation costs and potential regulatory hurdles, whereas the marginal costs of manufacturing are low. As discussed in previous chapters, increasing the number of different vial sizes would come at a cost. Each size is a different product from the manufacturer's perspective and raises the overall cost of production.

Regulatory guidance governing vial sharing varies among the U.S. Food and Drug Administration, the Centers for Medicare & Medicaid Services, the Centers for Disease Control and Prevention, and the

United States Pharmacopeia, and thus creates ambiguity and confusion for clinicians and health care administrators, although there is limited information about the safety of vial sharing.

Several technologies and clinical strategies show promise for reducing discarded drugs from single-dose vials but are not encouraged by current policies or are not feasible without reducing current practice-based constraints.

Vial sharing and other clinical practices such as dose banding and dose rounding are possible mechanisms for reducing discarded drug. For small clinics and hospitals, vial sharing may be challenging to coordinate due to limited patient volume as well as the need to obtain special equipment to allow prolonged storage for safe drug use.

RECOMMENDATION 2-2: The Secretary of the U.S. Department of Health and Human Services should direct the Centers for Medicare & Medicaid Services, the U.S. Food and Drug Administration, and the Centers for Disease Control and Prevention to work with the United States Pharmacopeia and other nonfederal partners, pharmacists, and infectious disease experts to review and harmonize existing policies and guidelines on drug administration and repackaging. These policies and guidelines should be informed by the successful experiences from other industrialized countries in reducing the amounts of discarded drugs.

RECOMMENDATION 4-1: The Secretary of the U.S. Department of Health and Human Services should direct the Centers for Medicare & Medicaid Services, the U.S. Food and Drug Administration, and the Centers for Disease Control and Prevention to initiate a partnership with other agencies, including the U.S. Department of Defense and the U.S. Department of Veterans Affairs, to work with health care and other organizations with expertise in areas such as industrial design and systems engineering to identify and implement technological systems that allow single-dose vials to be used safely across multiple patients.

RECOMMENDATION 4-2: The Secretary of the U.S. Department of Health and Human Services (HHS) should develop and implement policies that require drug manufacturers to produce injectable and infused drugs in multiple-dose vials when it is safe to do so. The Secretary of HHS should routinely review and evaluate the impact of such policies.

Goal 2: Implement an Efficient and Effective Reimbursement System for Clinician Administration of Infused or Injected Drugs

The biopharmaceutical supply chain, especially in the United States, contains numerous intermediaries who negotiate drug prices, establish the lists of drugs covered by insurance, and act as drug distributors, prescribers, and patients. For Medicare Part B, prescribers largely determine which drugs are to be purchased, and patient cost-sharing is specified by insurance plans. Medicare and private payers reimburse health care providers for the drugs they administer based on the drug's average sales price (ASP) plus a percentage add-on for administering the drug to account for costs incurred in drug delivery, mixing, and storage. Because the add-on is based on a percentage, the dollar amount is larger when the drug price is high. Thus, the reimbursement for the drug and the add-on may incentivize the selection and administration of higher cost drugs. Uncoupling the payments from the drug ASP, and focusing the payment for clinical administration on CMS's assessment of the time and complexity of treatment administration and safety monitoring would minimize incentives for clinicians' selection and administration of more expensive drugs when alternatives are available.

Accordingly, the concern about discarded drugs is partly due to the particular approach to paying—and reimbursing health care providers—for these drugs. Currently, under Medicare Part B, a clinician or health care provider (clinic, physician office, or hospital) typically buys drugs directly from manufacturers or from intermediaries, such as wholesalers or specialty pharmacies, stores them, and administers them to a patient as needed. The health care provider then submits a claim to the patient's health insurer for reimbursement, including for any drug that is discarded. The committee recognizes the importance of how changes to the current reimbursement for clinician-administered drugs would have a substantial impact, not only on health care providers but also on Medicare, private insurance payers, and patients, and that any actions toward that end may require modifications to existing law.

Under the current system in which drugs are developed, administered, or paid for, health care providers do not have incentives that encourage the efficient use of infused or injectable drugs in single-dose vials. They receive payment for up to the amount of drug indicated on the label of a single-dose vial, including that which is discarded. This lack of incentives could discourage efforts to reduce the amount of discarded drugs.

RECOMMENDATION 2-3: The Secretary of the U.S. Department of Health and Human Services should require the Centers for Medicare & Medicaid Services (CMS) to uncouple add-on payments to clinicians for infused or injected drugs under Medicare Part B from the drug average sales price, focusing the add-on payment instead on CMS's assessment of the time and complexity of drug management and safety monitoring.[2]

RECOMMENDATION 2-4: The Secretary of the U.S. Department of Health and Human Services should require the Center for Medicare & Medicaid Innovation to design and evaluate new payment models that reimburse health care providers by treatment episode, rather than by the volume or cost of a drug vial. Findings from the demonstrations should be disseminated widely to other relevant federal agencies, private payers, purchasers, clinicians, and consumers.

Currently, the JW modifier is the mechanism through which the discarded amount of drug from a single-dose vial is documented and reimbursed. As discussed in previous chapters, the very nature of administering single-dose drugs makes them prone to some portions being discarded. Medicare reimburses health care providers the amount of drug indicated on the vial or package label of a single-dose product, including what is discarded. The requirement for coding with the JW modifier appears to be an administrative burden for health care providers because the level of compliance is highly variable. Not all health care providers use the code, and those who do use it do so inconsistently. Some observers have argued that enforcing the requirement for using the JW modifier would lead to increased transparency regarding discarded drug payments. Others, however, argue that the JW modifier provides an economic incentive for discarding drugs and hinders efficient ways to distribute or administer drugs because it allows health care providers to be reimbursed regardless of whether all of the drug is actually used.

The committee recognizes that several analyses using data from the JW modifier have reported that the discarded drugs may be costing CMS billions of dollars annually. The estimates do not accurately capture the economic value of discarded drugs because they are based on the assumption that every ounce in a vial has an equal value and that the value of an ounce administered to treat a patient is equal to the value of an ounce of drug that is discarded, which, in reality, is not the case. As explained in

[2] The text in this recommendation was modified since the prepublication release of this report to improve technical accuracy of the language around payments to clinicians for infused or injected drugs under Medicare Part B.

previous chapters, it is easy enough to multiply the per-milliliter cost of a drug by the number of milliliters discarded each year to get a putative value for how much is "wasted" and then add up all such drugs to get a total, but interpreting that number as the value of the discarded drugs is problematic, given the decisions that go into pricing and reimbursing for these drugs in this country. The price of a drug is typically based not on how much is used but on the willingness to pay for the drug's therapeutic benefit. Put differently, because manufacturing costs do not drive drug prices, the quantity of a drug that a patient receives also does not drive pricing. Because of this, payment strategies used in many other countries provide a uniform reimbursement for a given treatment no matter how much of the drug was required for a specific patient.

Based on this assessment, as previously noted, the committee concludes that a significant amount of money cannot be recouped from discarded drugs to be used to offset federal health care costs. In essence, compliance with the JW requirement would enable CMS to track the amount of drug that is discarded from single-dose vials but does not offer practical ways to reduce the amount of discarded drugs.

Currently, attempting to estimate a single value for the cost of discarded drugs from single-dose vials to the Medicare program using the JW modifier would be incomplete and underestimated because the modifier is underused by health care providers and the resulting data may not be representative. Also, information on discarded drugs from Medicare Advantage plans and other commercial insurance plans are currently not available.

The use of the JW modifier as a basis for data collection and measurement of the amount of discarded drugs from single-dose vials has no current practical application to addressing the issue of discarded drugs under the current system in which drugs are developed, administered, or paid for.

RECOMMENDATION 3-1: While the current Medicare Part B drug reimbursement system is in place, the Centers for Medicare & Medicaid Services should discontinue the use of the JW modifier.

Several versions of draft congressional legislation focused on discarded drugs from single-dose drug vials have proposed rebates from manufacturers to health care providers and payers for discarded drug amounts. However, most bills do not propose refunds directed to patients, who would continue to have cost-sharing responsibilities for the cost of discarded drugs that were not used in their care.

Legislative initiatives proposing manufacturer rebates to providers and or payers for discarded drugs ignore the fact that a patient often would have been required to pay part of the cost of this discarded drug.

Based on the committee's assessment, it is not feasible to recoup significant funds via rebates for discarded drugs that could be spent on other health care services, so manufacturer rebates for unused drug are unlikely to achieve the intended aim. Also, given the variety of ways that drugs are priced and reimbursed, a rebate system for clinician-administered drugs would likely be quite complex. Because the committee's assessment shows that there is limited economic value to discarded drugs from single-dose vials under the current system in which drugs are developed, administered or paid for, a rebate strategy seems unlikely to achieve the intended goals. However, if the rebates that have been proposed in legislation are indeed implemented, the committee asserts that patients need to be included in those rebates.

RECOMMENDATION 4-3: In the event that legislation is enacted or regulatory action is taken to require rebates from manufacturers for discarded drugs, the U.S. Congress should require that rebates be directed first to cover the patient's out-of-pocket expense for the discarded drug and thereafter to health care providers and payers.

INTERDEPENDENCIES OF RECOMMENDATIONS

The nation's biopharmaceutical sector—including the researchers who develop and test drugs, drug manufacturers and distributors, pharmacies, the hospitals and health care providers who administer the drugs, the payers (such as Medicare and private health plans), and the various agencies that regulate drug development, manufacture, use, and reimbursement—is a complex, interconnected system. Changes in one part of the system inevitably affect other parts, often in unanticipated or even undesirable ways. Those looking to implement the recommendations in the report should keep this in mind and be aware of how a proposed change in one area may also affect other areas.

Policy makers should also note that this report's recommendations are interdependent, although their interrelationships vary. In some cases, two or more recommendations are designed to have similar effects, such as the multiple recommendations intended to move the system away from the current standard practice of discarding whatever drug is left in a vial after a single patient has been treated rather than sharing the vial among patients. In other cases, recommendations may focus on different issues. The ultimate goal of Recommendation 2-4, for instance, is to create a more equitable payment system. The committee recognizes that different people may have different goals in achieving an equitable payment system, including all patients paying the same amount for the same treatment or payment based on need, ability to pay, or to ensure that the needs of the most vulnerable are first addressed. If this goal is met, Recommendation 4-3 may not be necessary. But until that payment system is achieved, the recommendation to cover patients' out-of-pocket expenses with manufacturer rebates is intended to keep the system as fair as possible, so that patients are billed only for the amount of drug they receive and not also for the amount of leftover drug in a vial—the current system charges patients based on a factor totally unrelated to the patient (the size of the vial in which the manufacturer has chosen to package the drug) (see Figure 6-1).

Also, consider Recommendations 2-1 and 4-2. Both strive to promote the effective use of infused or injectable drugs in efficient and safe ways but feature different approaches. The ultimate goal of Recommendation 2-1 is to reduce the proportions of the content of vials that are discarded. Fixed doses reduce the proportion of drugs that are discarded but would not completely eliminate leftover drug. For example, in the case where different amounts of fixed doses are used for different indications of a drug that is available only in a vial that is sized for one of those indications, some drug may still be discarded. However, weight-based dosing results in a wide range in doses and amount of drug needed per patient. Consequently, it is almost certain that there will be remaining drug in the vial. The goal of Recommendation 4-2 is to reduce the proportions of drugs discarded by allowing the content of a vial to be used for more than one patient. If this recommendation is implemented, Recommendation 2-1 may not be necessary.

Policy makers need to be aware of and prepared for the possibility of unintended consequences of implementing new policies. For example, as long as drug manufacturers have near-total freedom to set drug prices, they will likely react to policies that reduce their profits. Thus if Recommendation 4-3 is adopted, and rebates from manufacturers for discarded drugs are directed to patients to cover their out-of-pocket expense, manufacturers may respond by increasing the price of individual vials so that the profit margins they realize from a particular drug remain approximately the same. Another potential unintended consequence is that the widespread use of multiple-dose vials envisioned in Recommendation 4-2 could give an advantage to larger medical centers, where there are more likely to be multiple patients who need the same drug at approximately the same time and thus can jointly receive the contents of a multi-dose vial. Smaller centers would be less likely to benefit due to vials' expiration between recipients.

While the committee's recommendations aim to achieve greater efficiencies in the manufacturing, distribution, and use of injected or infused

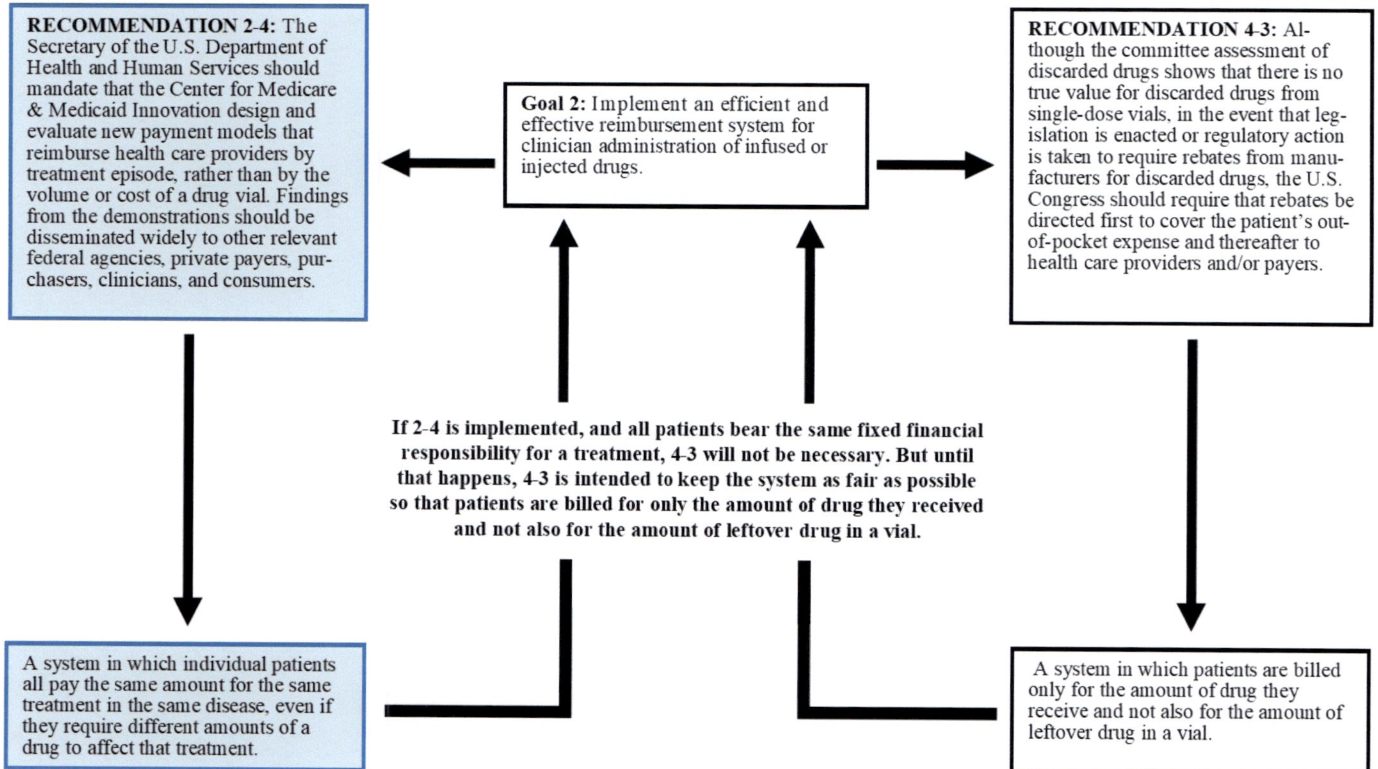

FIGURE 6-1 A representation of how two recommendations focus on different issues but are intended to have similar effects by moving the system away from the current standard practice.

drugs, it is not possible to predict how much, if any, financial savings might be associated with implementing those recommendations in the absence of additional data for economic analyses. The case for these recommendations is based mainly on nonfinancial considerations, such as safety and equity and overall efficiency.

The Pervasive Issue of Drug Pricing

As discussed in previous chapters, the issue of discarded weight-based drugs from single-dose vials takes place in the larger context of concerns about skyrocketing drug prices in the country. One of the clearest lessons from this investigation into weight-based drugs is the burden that the cost of such drugs places on many patients who rely on them to extend or save their lives. Regardless of whether some portion of a drug vial is discarded, many of these drugs are very expensive—thousands of dollars per treatment is not unusual—and traditional fee-for-service Medicare beneficiaries pay up to 20 percent of the billed amount for their medical care, without a cap on annual expenses. Supplemental private insurance and, in some cases, Medicaid can reduce out-of-pocket costs significantly, although that burden may not be totally eliminated.

> ***Concerns about reducing discarded drug take place in the larger context of concerns about drug costs, and particularly the cost to patients, in the United States.***
>
> ***Under the current system in which drugs are developed, administered or paid for, approaches to reduce the discarding of drugs from single-dose vials could have unintended consequences. Successful efforts may eventually trigger drug companies to raise the prices to derive constant or increased revenue for their products. Approaches to reducing discarded drugs from single-dose vials would need to leverage other strategies aimed at lowering drug prices, including allowing the Secretary of the U.S. Department of Health and Human Services to negotiate directly with manufacturers regarding the price of drugs.***

It is important to emphasize the connection between discarded drugs from single-dose vials and the resulting economic hardship for many Americans due to the prices of these expensive drugs. The high costs of U.S. prescription drugs are particularly burdensome for older Americans in the Medicare population—individuals who often have multiple chronic conditions, such as cancer, rheumatoid arthritis, and other immune disorders—and for individuals who are unfortunate enough to develop a disease whose treatment requires more expensive drugs. Among Medicare beneficiaries, those without supplemental insurance incur substantially higher out-of-pocket costs than their counterparts with private or other supplemental coverage. Even for those individuals with health insurance, most have deductibles, copayments, or coinsurance to pay.

The 2018 National Academies of Sciences, Engineering, and Medicine report *Making Medicines Affordable: A National Imperative* put forward a range of proposals to help prevent drug expenditures from spiraling out of control without discouraging continued innovation in drug development. This committee endorses the proposals in that report. In Chapter 5, the committee described how allowing the Secretary of the U.S. Department of Health and Human Services to negotiate directly for drugs could reduce the overall spending on Part B drugs for Medicare and for patients. This committee recognizes the importance of that proposal to reduce drug prices and to guard against unintended consequences in efforts to reduce discarded drugs and the associated costs, and it also recognizes that allowing the secretary to negotiate directly would require modifications to the Medicare Modernization Act of 2003 prohibiting the Medicare program from negotiating the price of drugs with manufacturers. In short, the set of recommendations offered in this report would yield significant results if they are leveraged with these other broader strategies aimed at lowering drug prices in the United States.

A PIVOTAL TIME FOR ACTION

Ideally, implementing these recommendations would lead to a future in which the development, use, and payment for weight-based drugs look different in a number of ways. First, fewer drugs would be administered based on weight. While there may always be certain drugs that are best administered in doses based on weight, BSA, or some related patient characteristic, many of the weight-based drugs being used today would likely work just as well with fixed doses, eliminating the need to calculate the dose by a patient's weight. The general assumption in oncology that drugs should be administered according to weight needs to be challenged, so that only those drugs that truly require it are developed and studied in trials as weight-based drugs.

For those drugs that do require weight-based dosing, the ideal future will be one in which multiple-use vials are much more common, minimizing the amounts of these expensive drugs that must be discarded. To the extent that there still is a need for vials smaller than today's single-dose vials, ideally, these should also be designed and manufactured, or managed using new technologies (Recommendation 4-1), so that they can be used by more than one patient.

Finally, in the ideal future, payments for weight-based drugs will be more fair than they are today and drugs more affordable for all patients who need them. Moving away from payments based on the amount of drug used and toward episode-based payments will make the system more fair and more manageable, but the recommendations here can do relatively little to make drugs more affordable. Uncoupling physician payments for administration from drug price (Recommendation 2-3) will remove one incentive for physicians to use more expensive drugs. Ultimately, ensuring drug affordability will require a much broader and more sustained effort, of the sort described in the *Making Medicines Affordable* report, which is why Chapter 5 of this report reiterates some of the recommendations from that study.

The United States needs to act now more than ever due to an aging society and other factors, including the rising cost of health care.

Appendix A

Glossary

The definitions marked with an asterisk are from the glossary included in the 2018 National Academies of Sciences, Engineering, and Medicine report *Making Medicines Affordable: A National Imperative.*

Average sales price (ASP)*—The ASP is derived from the manufacturer's unit sales of a drug to all U.S. purchasers in a calendar quarter divided by the number of units sold, after all discounts and rebates (except Medicaid rebates).

Beyond use date—Typically assigned to pharmacy compounded preparations to indicate the date after which a compounded preparation shall not be used, it is set based on the date on which the preparation was compounded.

Biological products (biologics)*—A category of products regulated by the U.S. Food and Drug Administration, including vaccines, blood and blood components, allergenic compounds, somatic cells, gene therapy, tissues, and recombinant therapeutic proteins.

Biosimilar—A biological drug that is very much like another biological drug (called the reference drug) that has already been approved by the U.S. Food and Drug Administration. Biosimilar drugs and reference drugs are made from living organisms, but they may be made in different ways and of slightly different substances.

Body surface area–based dosing—Drug dosing based on calculations made from height and weight together.

Clinical trial*—A formal study carried out according to a prospectively defined protocol that is intended to discover or verify the safety and the effectiveness of procedures or interventions in humans.

Clinician-administered drug—An outpatient drug other than a vaccine that is typically administered by infusion or injection by a health care provider in a physician's office or other outpatient clinical setting.

Closed-system transfer devices—Systems that include multiple components that are used in various combinations when moving a drug from one container to another.

Coinsurance*—The percentage of costs of a covered health care service that a beneficiary will pay after a deductible has been met.

Copay*—A fixed amount that a beneficiary will pay for a covered health care service after the deductible has been met.

Cost-sharing*—The share of costs covered by a beneficiary's insurance that he or she will pay out of pocket. This term generally includes deductibles, coinsurance, and copayments or similar charges, but it does not include premiums, balance billing amounts for non-network providers, or the cost of non-covered services.

Deductible*—The amount a beneficiary will pay for covered health care services before the insurance plan starts to pay.

Dose banding —A dosing method that standardizes injectable drugs into a defined set of dose ranges for patients.

Dose capping—A dosing method similar to dose rounding that is specifically designed to increase patient safety in obese populations.

Dose rounding—A dosing method that either increases or decreases a prescribed dose to the nearest whole vial strength available.

Drug repackaging—The act of dividing the content of a vial from the container in which it was distributed by the original manufacturer into multiple individual-dose containers without further manipulation of the drug. It also includes placing the contents of multiple containers of the same finished drug product into one container, as long as the container does not include other ingredients.

Expiration date—The date before which a drug manufacturer will guarantee the potency and safety of the drug content when stored in the recommended conditions and in the original container.

Federally qualified health centers—Community-based health care providers that receive funds from the Health Resources and Services Administration Health Center Program to provide primary care services in underserved areas.

Fee-for-service system—A system of health insurance payment in which health care providers are reimbursed for each particular service rendered on the basis of the number of services they provide.

Fixed dosing—Also known as flat dosing, refers to dosing strategies that do not take into account body size or other pharmacological parameters.

Formulary*—An approved list of medications that may be prescribed for a particular hospital, health system, health insurance policy, or pharmacy benefit.

Integrated health care delivery system—A network of health care providers that coordinates a continuum of services to a defined population and is typically held clinically and fiscally accountable for the outcomes and health status of the population served.

List price*—The prices that purchasers display as those at which they are prepared to sell their products and/or the prices regulated by legislation.

Multiple-dose vial—A vial that is intended to contain more than one dose of a drug and is intended to be administered multiple times and for multiple patients.

Out-of-pocket costs*—The expenses for medical care that are not reimbursed by insurance and are the responsibility of the beneficiary to pay. Out-of-pocket costs include deductibles, coinsurance, and copayments for covered services plus all costs for services that are not covered.

Pivotal trial—Also referred to as pivotal study, it is a clinical trial or study that intends to provide the ultimate evidence and data that the U.S. Food and Drug Administration uses to decide whether to approve a potential new medicine.

Rebate*—A payment made to a purchaser after the transaction has occurred.

Single-dose vial—A vial that is intended to contain one dose of a drug and to be used a single time for a single patient.

Specialty drugs—A general term for medications that have one or more of the following characteristics: are highly expensive, are molecularly complex (often derived from living cells), have limited availability or are available only through a specialized distribution network, have unique storage or shipment requirements, or are used for treating rare and complex disease indications.

Vial sharing—The practice of using residual drug from a vial to treat other patients within an acceptable time frame.

Waste—For efficiency in health care spending, waste refers to any spending that does not produce as much value as it could have if it were directed differently. This waste can appear in a variety of forms: administrative waste (e.g., excess overhead costs), operational waste (e.g., duplication of services), and clinical waste (e.g., practices that do not improve health outcomes or are detrimental to the patient). For the purposes of this report, the committee understood waste to generally refer to the discarded portions of weight-based drugs contained in single-dose vials.

Weight-based dosing—Drug dosing based on measures of "body size," including both dosing based on weight and dosing based on body surface area, which is based on calculations made from weight and height together.

Wholesalers*—Drug distribution companies that purchase drugs from the manufacturers and then sell them to pharmacies at negotiated prices.

Appendix B

Supplemental Figures and Tables from Commissioned Analyses

As described in Chapter 3, the committee commissioned two analyses to understand the extent of health care costs—to the Medicare program, to private health care payers, and to patients—that arise from billing for discarded drugs and biologicals from single-dose vials. The focus of these analyses was not to assess the economic value of the discarded drug but rather to get a sense of the amount of drugs that are being discarded and to identify any inefficiencies in the current system of tracking the amount of discarded drugs yearly. One analysis looked at Medicare claims that used the JW modifier code,[1] examining how much of total Medicare spending they represent; examined patterns in the claims using the JW modifier code and whether those claims accurately reflected the amount spent each year by Medicare on discarded drugs; and explored compliance with the JW modifier. The second analysis looked at the use of the JW modifier in the private health care system and estimated the costs associated with discarded drugs for both patients and their payers in this system.

The key findings from those two analyses are described in Chapter 3, but the analyses included a great many results and details that were not included in the chapter. These additional results are provided below in

[1] As described in Chapters 2 and 3, the JW modifier is the mechanism through which health care providers can bill and be reimbursed for the discarded portion of a drug from a single-dose vial in a way that formally documents the amount of drug that was discarded. The modifier can be used for any single-dose vial in which some drug is discarded, regardless of whether the drug is administered in a fixed dose or a dose based on weight.

the form of figures and tables describing the use of the JW modifier in various situations and settings.

COSTS OF DISCARDED DRUGS

The first issue the researchers addressed was the insurance payment associated with the portion of drugs discarded each year, both drugs that are paid for by Medicare and those paid for by private insurers. Basic estimates of payment for the discarded drugs can be obtained by adding up the payment of the drug claims for which the JW modifier was applied. However, given the evidence of inconsistent use of the JW modifier by physicians (described in Chapter 3), it is likely that a significant percentage of discarded drugs are never reported via the JW modifier, implying that the estimates of the total payment of discarded drugs based on Medicare claims are likely to be significantly low. Thus, the researchers went beyond these basic calculations to obtain a more accurate idea of the amount of spending on the drugs that are discarded each year.

For example, to get a sense of just how low the JW modifier–based estimates of waste are for drugs paid for by Medicare Part B, the researchers analyzed the top five drugs in terms of spending on discarded drugs (i.e., spending associated with claims with the JW modifier) and estimated the amount of spending on discarded drugs that was not reported. This was done by first calculating a patient-drug-specific ratio of JW-associated spending to total spending for claims with the JW modifier and then applying that ratio to calculate additional potential waste for observed encounters where the patient received the drug but there was no claim for discarded drug (i.e., claim with the JW modifier) for that encounter. As shown in Table B-1, the total spending on discarded drug as a percentage of total spending for the drug ranged from 9 percent to 27 percent for these drugs without accounting for the amount of unreported spending. After including the estimated amount of unreported spending on discarded drugs, the percentage ranged from 11 percent to 28 percent. It is important to note that even with the inclusion of the estimated unreported spending, these figures are likely an underestimation of spending on discarded drug because it is not possible to calculate potential waste for patient–drug combinations where the JW modifier was never used, which accounts for a sizable percentage of patient–drug combinations.

In another analysis to estimate the costs of discarded drugs, the researchers included only health care providers who used the JW modifier. Wide variations across drugs were also observed between calculation that included and excluded health care providers who never used the JW modifier (see Table B-2). In some drugs (e.g., omalizumab), the difference

TABLE B-1 Estimated Costs of Discarded Drugs Paid for by Medicare Part B ($ millions), 2018

Drug	Total Part B Spending ($ in millions)	Observed JW Waste Spending	Total Observed JW Waste Spending as a Percentage of Total Part B Spending (%)	Potential Waste Spending, Patient-Drug Level	Total Waste Spending (observed + potential)	Total Waste Spending as a Percentage of Total Part B Spending (%)
Bortezomib	90.5	24.2	27	1.31	25.51	28
Trastuzumab	175	15.9	9	4.20	20.10	11
Romiplostim	48.4	10.6	22	2.01	12.61	26
Paclitaxel Protein-Bound	56	7.6	14	1.05	8.61	15
Carfilzomib	52.1	6.7	13	1.41	8.13	16

NOTES: Top five drugs in terms of spending on claims with the JW modifier, 2018. All estimates based on the 20 percent sample and not scaled to estimate 100 percent.

TABLE B-2 Use of the JW Modifier and Associated Spending Among Medicare Part B Providers Who Sometimes/Always Used Modifier, 2018

	Excluding Health Care Providers Who Never Used JW Modifier		Including Health Care Providers Who Never Used JW Modifier	
	Percent of Claims with the JW Modifier	Percent of Spending on the JW Modifier Claims	Percent of Claims with the JW Modifier	Percent of Spending on the JW Modifier Claims
Belimumab	47.0	3.3	36.3	2.6
OnabotulinumtoxinA	54.9	11.6	36.3	7.9
Daptomycin	42.1	17.5	20.2	9.2
Decitabine	85.4	25.2	74.6	22.6
Golimumab	65.6	9.7	51.2	7.6
Infliximab	22.7	2.2	14.4	1.4
Omalizumab	45.3	10.3	25.2	6.3
Romiplostim	71.1	22.9	67.5	22.0
Tocilizumab	48.8	4.1	34.8	2.9
Azacitidine	84.4	24.6	76.4	22.8
Bortezomib	87.6	29.1	79.7	27.0
Brentuximab Vedotin	67.1	11.3	63.9	10.8
Cabazitaxel	90.1	28.5	85.3	27.2
Carfilzomib	75.4	14.2	68.7	12.9
Cetuximab	46.4	4.0	41.4	3.6
Daratumumab	37.6	1.7	33.0	1.5
Elotuzumab	46.8	5.1	38.8	4.2
Ipilimumab	56.9	8.4	54.0	8.0
Paclitaxel Protein-Bound	73.3	15.3	64.9	13.9
Panitumumab	57.8	6.2	52.7	5.7
Pemetrexed Disodium	51.1	3.3	44.8	2.9
Ramucirumab	59.2	4.5	55.2	4.2
Ado-Trastuzumab Emtansine	63.3	7.1	57.5	6.6
Trastuzumab	65.5	10.5	58.3	9.4
Doxorubicin HCL Peg-Liposomal	22.9	4.4	18.4	3.5

NOTES: Sample of drugs include those with greater than 10 percent claims with the JW modifier in 2018. Excluded health care providers with fewer than 11 claims for a given drug.

in the percentage spending on JW claims could be as large as 50 percent (i.e., 10.3 percent versus 6.3 percent).

The committee's second commissioned analysis examined the use of the JW modifier in drug treatments paid for by private insurers. Although the MarketScan data used in this analysis did not allow for the sorts of physician-to-physician comparisons that were carried out with the Medicare data, the consultant performed an analysis with patient–drug pairs (i.e., situations involving one patient being treated with the same drug on multiple occasions) to gain insight into how consistently the JW modifier is used in claims on private insurance. For each patient–drug pair the consultant categorized compliance with the Centers for Medicare & Medicaid Services (CMS) mandate of the JW modifier into three levels: no compliance, partial compliance, and full compliance.

Of the 62 drugs with at least one JW modifier claim, the researcher focused specifically on the 25 drugs for which there was at least a 5 percent JW compliance rate at the patient–drug pair level (see Table B-3). Of these, azacitidine had the highest JW compliance rate, with full compliance for 18.51 percent of patient–drug pairs and partial compliance for 23.51 percent of patient–drug pairs. A total of 17 drugs had a JW compliance rate of at least 20 percent when full and partial compliance rates were combined.

The researchers imputed the potential additional spending on discarded drugs using the same approach described in the Medicare analysis by applying a patient–drug-specific ratio to the partially compliant group. The researchers found that using the approach employed by CMS, discarded drugs accounted for 0.81 percent of total insurance payment on the 18 drugs with discarded amount over $1 million (see Table B-4). However, this percentage was based on the underused JW modifier. When the potential additional spending imputed from the partially compliant group was included, the percentage of total insurance payment on discarded drugs increased to 1.6 percent (see Table B-4). For some drugs the difference between imputed and raw percentage was large. For example, the raw percent was 3.9 percent for carfilzomib and the imputed percentage was close to 8 percent. This analysis again demonstrated the underestimation of costs associated with discarded drugs when the calculation was relying on the use of the JW modifier.

To better understand the financial impact of discarded drugs, the researchers conducted an additional analysis that used the actual weight and height of patients to determine the discarded percentage of their drugs. In the MarketScan data, there is Health Risk Assessment (HRA) survey data that include patients' self-reported weight and height information. From the 77 Part B drugs, the researchers identified 45 weight-based drugs. They abstracted recommended drug dosage and its vial size for a drug to treat a specific disease based on IBM Micromedex. They then

TABLE B-3 Distribution of Percentage of JW Compliance Among Drugs with at Least 5 Percent JW Modifier Claims in the MarketScan Data

		Number	Compliance (%)		
Drug	Generic Name	of Patients	No	Full	Partial
J9025	Azacitidine*	940	57.98	18.51	23.51
J1602	Golimumab	2,853	62.99	20.68	16.33
J9041	Bortezomib	3,640	64.2	17.17	18.63
J9043	Cabazitaxel	351	66.67	22.79	10.54
J0894	Decitabine*	545	67.16	18.35	14.5
J9047	Carfilzomib	1,005	68.76	10.05	21.19
J2796	Romiplostim	680	71.18	7.5	21.32
J9264	Paclitaxel Protein-Bound	3,678	71.83	14.11	14.06
J9354	Ado-Trastuzumab Emtansine	688	73.26	9.01	17.73
J0490	Belimumab	2,001	74.06	3.85	22.09
J3262	Tocilizumab	2,429	77.07	4.49	18.44
J9042	Brentuximab Vedotin	504	78.57	10.12	11.31
J9176	Elotuzumab	238	78.57	7.14	14.29
J9145	Daratumumab	1,182	78.6	4.23	17.17
J9305	Pemetrexed Disodium	3,844	78.85	8.82	12.33
J9355	Trastuzumab	9,925	78.89	3.85	17.26
J9308	Ramucirumab	824	79.85	8.62	11.53
J9055	Cetuximab	1,540	80.52	4.94	14.55
J0585	OnabotulinumtoxinA*	57,960	80.66	10.65	8.69
J9303	Panitumumab	738	81.17	5.15	13.69
J9228	Ipilimumab	1,378	81.71	10.3	7.98
J1745	Infliximab	28,552	89.14	2.52	8.35
Q2050	Doxorubicin HCL Peg-Liposomal*	1,946	92.24	1.95	5.81
J9299	Nivolumab	5,790	93.61	1.93	4.46
J0878	Daptomycin*	7,223	94.12	2.38	3.5

* Indicates multiple brand and/or generic names for a specific Healthcare Common Procedure Coding System code.

collected the drug claims of these 45 drugs from the Commercial Claims and Encounter databases and the Medicare Supplemental Databases in IBM MarketScan data in 2017. Then, they linked the HRA data with the drug claims to select patients with known weight/height; the final study cohort included 4,688 patients (see Figure B-1).

TABLE B-4 Percentage of JW Claims and Discarded Amount for 18 Drugs with Discarded Amount ≥ $1 Million in MarketScan Data

			Total		Percentage			
					JW Claim		JW Net Pay	
Generic	Observed Number of Claims	Number of Claims	Net Pay $ Million	JW Net Pay $ Million	Raw	Imputed	Raw	Imputed
Total	854,901	4,039,256	99,51.5	80.6	3.62	6.56	0.81	1.6
Trastuzumab	9,925	150,843	679	16	9.72	20.82	2.35	5.18
Infliximab	28,552	254,503	12,87.7	8.5	5.29	10.87	0.66	1.44
Bortezomib	3,640	98,359	121.1	7.3	18.18	27.09	6.06	8.79
OnabotulinumtoxinA*	57,960	219,057	183.5	7.1	13.29	20.28	3.89	5.69
Bevacizumab	38,194	228,783	489.9	5.9	4	8.11	1.2	2.47
Paclitaxel Protein-Bound	3,678	41,835	101	4.2	15.99	22.67	4.14	6.02
Ipilimumab	1,378	5,684	175.9	3.2	9.69	14.78	1.81	2.62
Carfilzomib	1,005	35,661	65.2	2.5	16.01	27.52	3.9	7.98
Golimumab	2,853	19,097	66.2	2.4	20.65	29.31	3.57	5.16
Brentuximab Vedotin	504	4,261	77.2	2.3	10.82	17.84	3.03	4.64
Romiplostim	680	20,427	43.4	2.3	16.05	29.7	5.33	9.92
Pembrolizumab	4,828	32,471	296.1	1.9	2.21	4.64	0.63	1.41
Ado-Trastuzumab Emtansine	688	8,367	66.1	1.7	13.1	24.51	2.56	4.87
Pemetrexed Disodium	3,844	26,535	139.2	1.6	10.97	20.37	1.17	2.16
Omalizumab	7,459	81,999	103.4	1.5	4.65	8.19	1.47	2.6
Cabazitaxel	351	2,391	14.7	1.1	20.16	24.97	7.37	9.83
Rituximab	17,568	87,867	584.7	1	0.68	1.85	0.18	0.56
Nivolumab	5,790	60,779	370.6	1	1.93	6.31	0.28	1.09

* Indicates multiple brand and/or generic names for a specific Healthcare Common Procedure Coding System code.

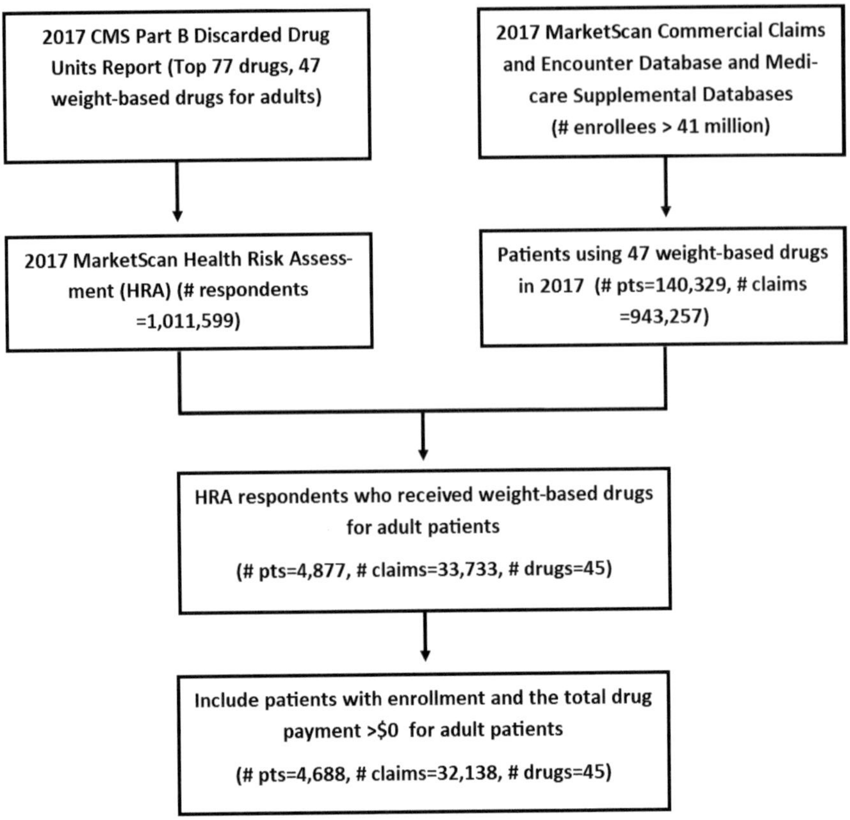

FIGURE B-1 Cohort ascertainment flowchart.
NOTE: CMS refers to the Centers for Medicare & Medicaid Services and pts refers to patients.

Of the 4,688 patients in the study cohort (see Figure B-7), the researchers multiplied patients' weight/height with recommended drug dosage to obtain patients' drug units used for treatment assuming no dose reduction, and computed the discarded drug units by subtracting patients' treatment drug units from the full vial sizes. They calculated the percentage of the discarded drug units by dividing the discarded units over the full vial sizes. They limited the analyses to drugs with more than 10 claims for each drug, and included 38 drugs. The findings are depicted in Figure B-2, which shows the mean, minimum, and maximum discarded percentage for each drug, ordered by the discarded percentages. The mean discarded percentage ranged from less than 1 percent to close to 40 percent. Furthermore, within each drug, variations in patients' weight

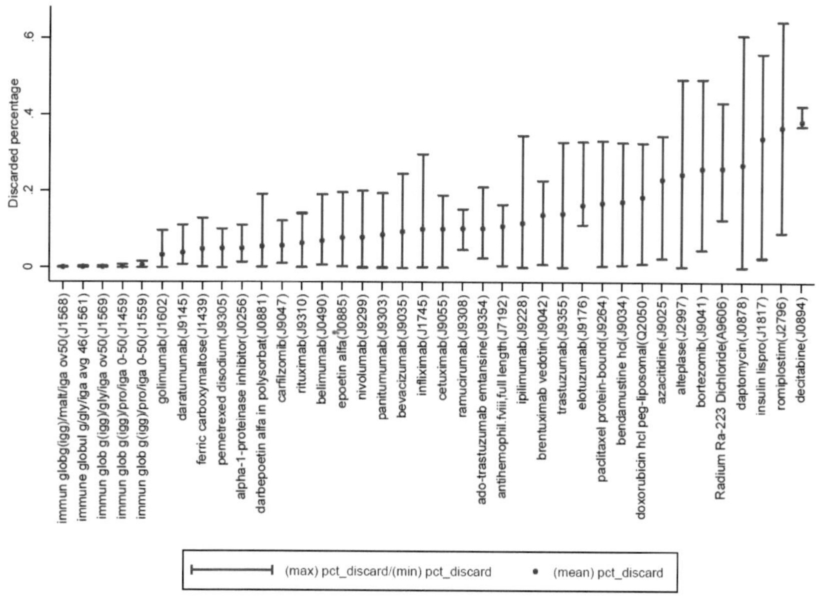

FIGURE B-2 Mean and maximum discarded units for 38 drugs based on patients' weight/height.

or BSA resulted in a noticeable range between minimum and maximum percentages for some drugs.

The researchers then analyzed payment variables from claims data to estimate the financial burden of discarded drugs for private payers and patients. On average, private insurance paid $36,652 per patient on weight-based drugs, and of this amount, $2,992 (8.2 percent) was spent on discarded drugs. The mean out-of-pocket cost was $1,043, and of this, $78 (7.5 percent) was spent on discarded drugs. Although the average out-of-pocket cost for discarded drugs was moderate, a small subset of patients disproportionately bore the financial burden, especially those enrolled in high-deductible plans. For these patients, the top 10 percent paid more than $380 for discarded drugs, whereas for patients not in high-deductible plans, the top 10 percent paid more than $260.

THE JW MODIFIER COMPLIANCE RATE

There was substantial variation in health care providers' use of the JW modifier from one drug to another, as shown in Figure B-3. To simplify this part of the analysis, the consultant restricted it to the 25 drugs in the

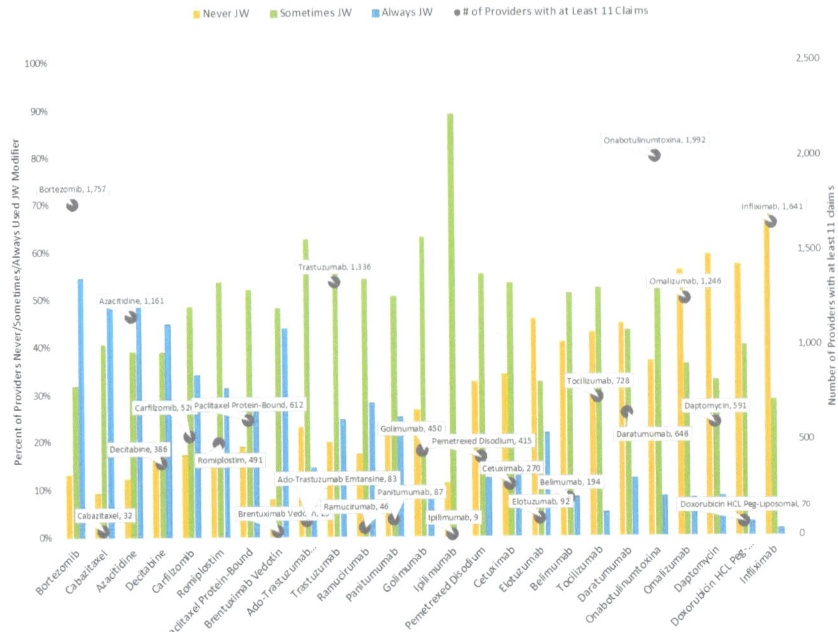

Notes: Analysis restricted to the 25 drugs with at least 10% claims with JW modifier. Drugs ranked by percent of claims with JW modifier.

FIGURE B-3 Percentage of health care providers' always/sometimes/never using the JW modifier for drugs with at least 10 percent claims with the JW modifier, 2018.

sample for which at least 10 percent of claims had the JW modifier and also restricted it to health care providers with at least 11 claims for the drug using a 20 percent random sample of Medicare fee-for-service outpatient and carrier claims in 2018. As the figure shows (y-axis), the number of health care providers included in the analysis varied widely according to the particular drug, from 9 health care providers with at least 11 claims for ipilimumab to close to 2,000 health providers with at least 11 claims for onabotulinumtoxinA. Among this sample of health care providers, the percentage who never used the JW modifier varied across drugs, from 8 percent of health care providers administering brentuximab vedotin never using the modifier for that drug to 70 percent of those administering infliximab. Given the large percentages of physicians with more than 11 claims who used the modifier in some cases but not others, there is clear evidence that health care providers' use of the JW modifier is inconsistent from one drug to another.

In addition to their analyses of spending on discarded drugs, the consultants who performed the Medicare analysis also looked for what factors might influence the likelihood that a physician will use the JW modifier. For example, to assess whether there was any relationship between the total amount Medicare spent on a drug and the likelihood that the JW modifier would be used in a claim, the researchers examined the percentage of claims with the JW modifier across drugs with different total allowed amounts in 2018. As shown in Figure B-4, there was very low negative correlation between total Medicare spending on a drug and the percentage of claims with the JW modifier.

A second possible correlation examined by the researchers was the influence of geographic region on likelihood of JW modifier use. Among weight-based drugs in the sample for which at least 1 percent of claims had the JW modifier (40 of 77 drugs), the researchers found few consistent patterns or substantial differences in terms of use of the modifier across regions, as shown in Figure B-5.

Nor was a physician's location in an urban versus a rural area a major factor in the use of the JW modifier. As shown in Figure B-6, among drugs in the sample for which at least 1 percent of Medicare claims had the JW modifier (40 of 77 drugs), the use of the JW modifier in urban versus rural areas did not follow any sort of consistent pattern.

As shown in Figure B-7, the rates of JW modifier use were similar between health care providers with above median number of claims for a particular drug (dark blue bars) and those with below the median number of claims (light blue bars) and also between health care providers in the bottom 25th (dark green bars) and top 25th percentiles (light green bars) of claims for that drug. There was no relationship between provider volume of claims and use of the JW modifier.

The only consistent pattern identified across drugs was the higher use of the JW modifier in physician office settings relative to hospital outpatient departments, as shown in Figure B-8. Across the 40 drugs in

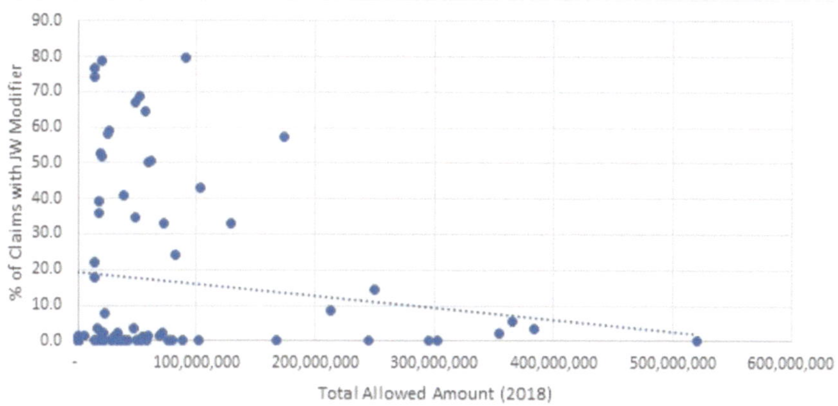

FIGURE B-4 Correlation between allowed amount and JW modifier use, 2018.

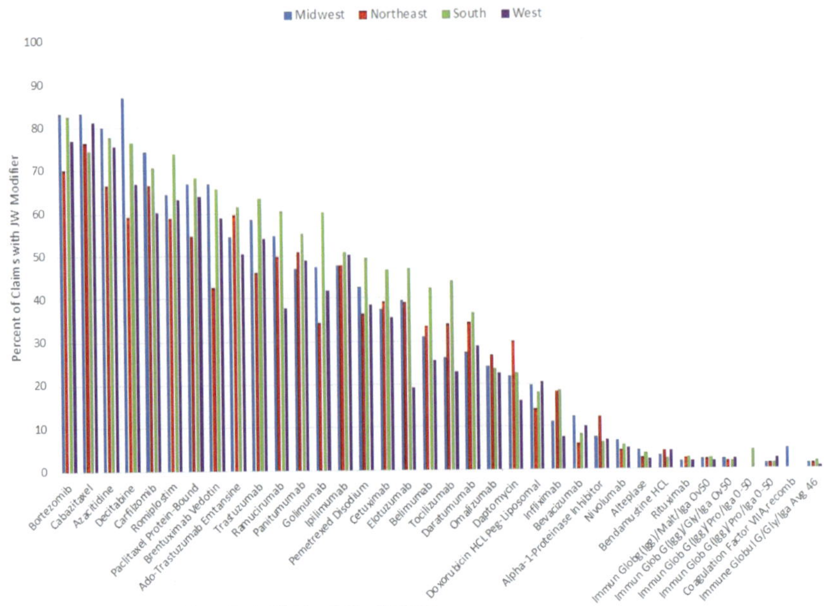

Notes: Sample for graph is weight-based drugs with at least 1% claims with JW modifier (N=36).

FIGURE B-5 Percentage of claims with the JW modifier for weight-based drugs with at least 1 percent of claims with the JW modifier by region, 2018.

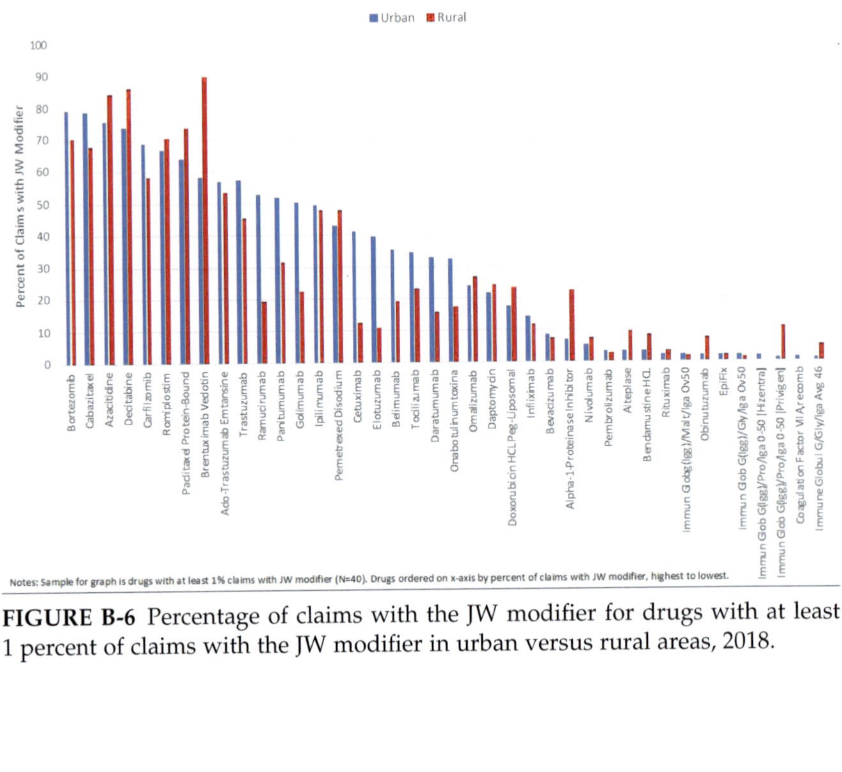

Notes: Sample for graph is drugs with at least 1% claims with JW modifier (N=40). Drugs ordered on x-axis by percent of claims with JW modifier, highest to lowest.

FIGURE B-6 Percentage of claims with the JW modifier for drugs with at least 1 percent of claims with the JW modifier in urban versus rural areas, 2018.

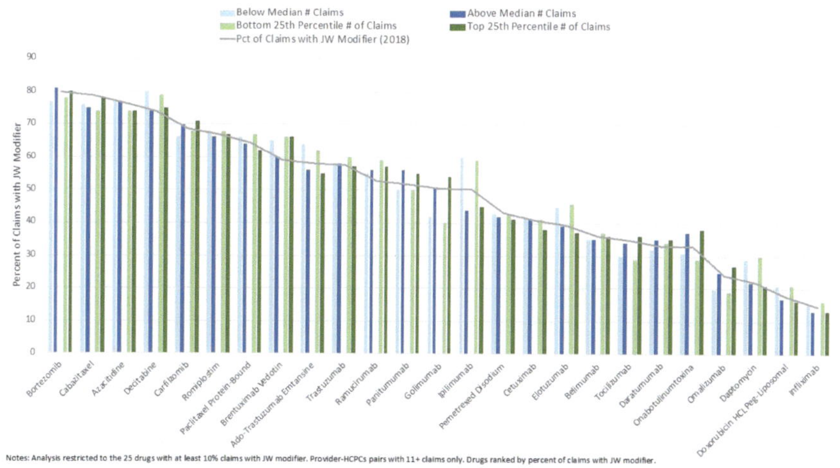

FIGURE B-7 Percentage of claims with the JW modifier for top waste drugs, by provider volume, 2018.

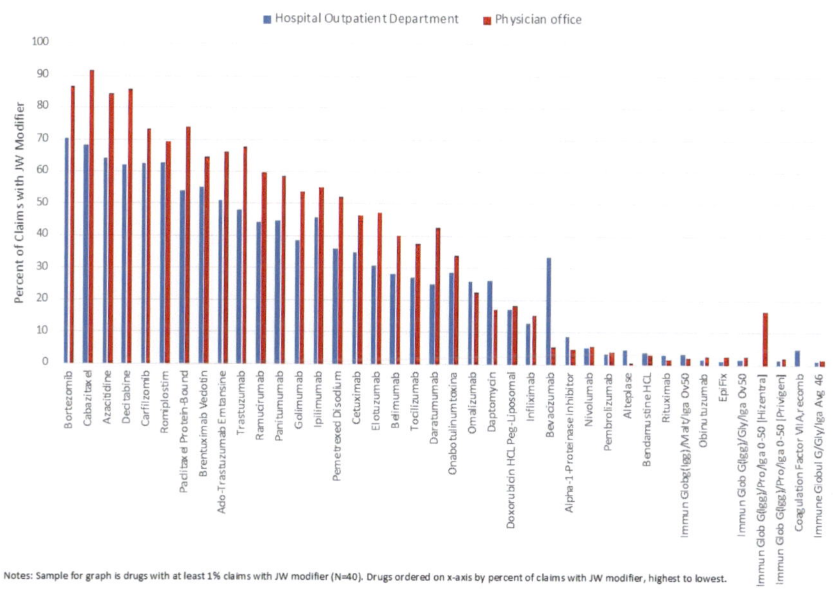

FIGURE B-8 Percentage of claims with the JW modifier for drugs with at least 1 percent of claims with the JW modifier by care setting, 2018.

the sample with at least 1 percent of Medicare claims with the JW modifier, JW modifier use was higher in terms of the percentage of claims for a given drug with the JW modifier in physician office settings relative to hospital outpatient departments.

Appendix C

Stakeholder Input

CORINNE AXELROD, Centers for Medicare & Medicaid Services
PETER BACH, Memorial Sloan Kettering Cancer Center
ALEXANDER BASTIAN, Value and Market Access Galapagos NV
CORBIN BENNETT, Kaiser Permanente
DONALD BERWICK, Institute for Healthcare Improvement
AMITABH CHANDRA, Harvard Kennedy School of Government
JACQUELINE CORRIGAN-CURAY, Office of Medical Policy, Center for Drug Evaluation and Research
JAY CROSSON, Kaiser Permanente
GWEN DARIEN, Patient Advocate Foundation
STACEY DUSETZINA, Vanderbilt University Medical Center
MICHAEL GANIO, ASHP Office of Practice Advancement
PETER GILBAR, University of Queensland
SHERRY GLIED, New York University
KEDAR GOKHALE, Janssen Research & Development Biotherapeutics on behalf of BioPhorum Fill Finish Group
DANIEL GOLDSTEIN, Petach Tkvah
MIREILLE JACOBSON, Center for Health Policy and Economics
RONALD KHOURY, U.S. Department of Defense
SARA LEVIN, House Committee on Ways and Means
PRABATH MALLUWA-WADU, Centers for Medicare & Medicaid Services
RICHARD L. SCILSKY, American Society of Clinical Oncology
MICHAEL SEIDEN, The US Oncology Network
BRIAN SERUMAGA, United States Pharmacopeia
SARAH SHIREY-LOSSO, Centers for Medicare & Medicaid Services

The committee also received written comments on the study from Cigna and BioPhorum. The comments are available in the public access file of the Committee on Implications of Discarded Weight-Based Drugs.

Appendix D

Biographical Information

Edward Shortliffe, M.D., Ph.D. (*Chair*), is the chair emeritus and an adjunct professor of biomedical informatics at Columbia University. He serves as an adjunct professor of biomedical informatics at Arizona State University and is also an adjunct professor of population health sciences at Weill Cornell Medical College. He has served as the president and the chief executive officer of the American Medical Informatics Association, a professor in the School of Biomedical Informatics at the University of Texas Health Science Center in Houston, a professor of biomedical informatics at Arizona State University, a professor of basic medical sciences and a professor of medicine at the University of Arizona College of Medicine, and the founding dean of the Phoenix campus of the University of Arizona's College of Medicine. He was the Rolf A. Scholdager Professor and the chair of the Department of Biomedical Informatics at the Columbia College of Physicians and Surgeons in New York City and a professor of medicine and computer science at Stanford University. He is a master of the American College of Physicians and was a member of that organization's board of regents. He is the editor-in-chief of the *Journal of Biomedical Informatics*. A recipient of several awards including a research career development award from the National Library of Medicine, the Grace Murray Hopper Award of the Association for Computing Machinery, and the Morris F. Collen Award of the American College of Medical Informatics, he was also appointed as a Henry J. Kaiser Family Foundation Faculty Scholar in General Internal Medicine. His research interests include the broad range of issues related to integrated decision-support systems, their effective implementation, and the role of the

Internet in health care. He received an A.B. in applied mathematics from Harvard College and both a Ph.D. in medical information sciences and an M.D. from Stanford University. An elected member of the American Society for Clinical Investigation, the Association of American Physicians, and the American Clinical and Climatological Association, he has also been elected to fellowship in the American College of Medical Informatics and the American Association for Artificial Intelligence. He is a member of the National Academy of Medicine.

Julie Donohue, Ph.D., is the vice chair for research and the co-director of the Ph.D. program in the Department of Health Policy and Management in the Graduate School of Public Health at the University of Pittsburgh. She directs the Medicaid Research Center, which provides analytic support to Pennsylvania's Medicaid program, and co-directs the Center for Pharmaceutical Policy and Prescribing. She conducts research on insurance coverage, financing, and delivery of health care with a focus on behavioral health care and pharmaceuticals. Her pharmaceutical policy work has informed both Medicare and Medicaid policy. Together with AcademyHealth, she recently launched the Medicaid Outcomes Distributed Research Network to support state Medicaid policy evaluations. She holds secondary appointments in the Clinical and Translational Science Institute and is a faculty affiliate in the Health Policy Institute. She earned a Ph.D. in health policy from Harvard University and completed a postdoctoral fellowship in pharmaceutical policy research at Harvard Medical School.

Anupam Jena, M.D., Ph.D., is the Ruth L. Newhouse Associate Professor of Health Care Policy at Harvard Medical School and a physician in the Department of Medicine at Massachusetts General Hospital. He is also a faculty research fellow at the National Bureau of Economic Research. His research involves several areas of health economics and policy, including the economics of physician behavior and the physician workforce, medical malpractice, the economics of health care productivity, and the economics of medical innovation. Dr. Jena provided compensated expert litigation consulting services in 2020 and 2021 to pharmaceutical companies including Merck, Genentech, Sanofi-Aventis, Janssen, and others through his affiliation with Analysis Group. Prior to his service on the committee, he was a consultant for pharmaceutical companies including Amgen, Eisai, and Otsuka through his affiliation with Precision Health Economics. He is a recipient of the Eugene Garfield Award from Research America for his work demonstrating the economic value of medical innovation in HIV/AIDS. He is a recipient of the National Institutes of Health's Director's Early Independence Award to fund research on the physician determinants of health care spending, quality, and patient outcomes and the International Society for Pharmacoeconomics and Outcomes Research New Investigator Award. He received his M.D. and Ph.D. in economics from the University of Chicago. He completed his residency in internal medicine at Massachusetts General Hospital. He served on the National Academies of Sciences, Engineering, and Medicine ad hoc Committee on Diagnostic Error in Health Care.[1]

Tracy Lieu, M.D., M.P.H., is the director of the Division of Research at Kaiser Permanente Northern California. She leads a department of 600 people who conduct studies in clinical effectiveness, delivery science, and epidemiology to benefit Kaiser Permanente members and society at large. She is also a practicing pediatrician who has led internationally recognized research in vaccine safety and policy and childhood asthma. Before her current role, she was a professor and a center director in the Department of Population Medicine at the Harvard Pilgrim Health Care Institute and Harvard Medical School. Her national roles have included membership on the U.S. Preventive Services Task Force and the Advisory Committee on Immunization Practices and the chair of the Health Services Organization and Delivery study section of the National Institutes of Health. She was elected to the National Academy of Medicine for her use of decision sciences and economic evaluation to inform health policy.

Gary Lyman, M.D., M.P.H., serves as a senior lead for health care quality and policy within the Hutchinson Institute for Cancer Outcomes Research at the Fred Hutchinson Cancer Research Center and as a professor of medicine, public health, and pharmacy at the University of Washington. He is a board-certified medical oncologist, hematologist, and public health researcher who focuses on comparative effectiveness, health technology assessment, and health services and outcomes research. He has served as an advisor to the U.S. Food and Drug Administration's Oncologic Drug Advisory Committee, and has been active in the Alliance for Clinical Trials in Oncology (formerly Cancer and Leukemia Group B), the SWOG Cancer Research Network, and the Eastern Cooperative Oncology Group. He has served on the Breast Cancer Screening and Diagnosis Panel and the Growth Factors Panel for the National Comprehensive Cancer Network and chairs clinical practice guidelines for the American Society of Clinical

[1] Anupam Jena's biosketch has been updated since the release of this report to disclose compensated expert litigation consulting services to pharmaceutical companies during the course of the study and other consulting services to pharmaceutical companies before the start of the study.

Oncology (ASCO) and the American Society of Hematology. He was the chief of medicine at the Moffitt Cancer Center and Research Institute and a professor of medicine at the University of South Florida, the University of Rochester, and Duke University. Additionally, he holds leadership positions within ASCO as well as the SWOG Cancer Research Network, for which he serves as the executive officer for cancer care delivery, symptom management and quality of life research, and immunotherapy. Dr. Lyman made invited presentations in 2020 regarding the ASCO clinical practice guidelines for complications of cancer chemotherapy, the development of clinical pathways in oncology, and the work of the ASCO taskforce on biosimilars for which he received compensation from Jazz Pharmaceuticals, Merck Sharp & Dohme, Partner Therapeutics, Sandoz, and Seagen. He earned his M.D. from the State University of New York and an M.P.H. in biostatistics from the Harvard T.H. Chan School of Public Health and pursued postdoctoral training at the Roswell Park Cancer Center and Dana-Farber Cancer Institute.[2]

Kavita Patel, M.D., M.P.H., is a non-resident fellow at the Brookings Institution and a primary care physician in Washington, DC. She advises health care technology and services organizations through New Enterprise Associates. She is a member of the U.S. Department of Health and Human Services Physician Focused Payment Model Technical Advisory Committee. Previously, she consulted for biopharmaceutical companies, directed the health policy program at the New America Foundation, and served in the Obama administration as the director of policy for the Office of Intergovernmental Affairs and Public Engagement in the White House. She is a practicing physician with health care policy experience in the U.S. Senate Health, Education, Labor, and Pensions Committee, where she was the deputy staff director for health under Senator Edward Kennedy. She was selected as a young global leader by the World Economic Forum and is a Society of General Internal Medicine advisory board member for the National Commission on Physician Payment Reform. She received her M.P.H. from the University of California, Los Angeles, and her M.D. from the University of Texas Health Science Center.

Harold Paz, M.D., M.S., is the executive vice president and the chancellor for health affairs at The Ohio State University and the chief executive officer of The Ohio State Wexner Medical Center. Before joining Ohio State in June 2019, he was the executive vice president and the chief

[2] Gary Lyman's biosketch has been updated since the release of this report to disclose compensated invited presentations to pharmaceutical companies made during the course of the study.

medical officer at CVS Health/Aetna, where he led clinical strategy and policy at the intersection of all of Aetna's domestic and global businesses. He reported to Aetna's chairman and chief executive officer and was a member of its executive committee. He was also an adjunct professor of internal medicine at the Yale University School of Medicine. Prior to joining Aetna, he served as the president and the chief executive officer of the Penn State Hershey Health System and as the senior vice president for health affairs at The Pennsylvania State University and the dean of its College of Medicine for 8 years. Before his appointment at Penn State, he spent 11 years as the dean of the Robert Wood Johnson Medical School and the chief executive officer of the Robert Wood Johnson University Medical Group. He is a fellow of the American College of Physicians and the American College of Chest Physicians. He is currently on the board of Research America and the advisory board of United Surgical Partners International. He is the past chair of the board of directors of the Association of Academic Health Centers and a former board member of the Association of American Medical Colleges (AAMC) and chair of the AAMC council of deans. He has served on a number of corporate and scientific boards in the health care and biotechnology field. He received his bachelor's degree from the University of Rochester, a master of science in life science engineering from Tufts University and his M.D. from the University of Rochester School of Medicine and Dentistry. He completed his residency at Northwestern University, where he served as the chief medical resident. He was a Eudowood Fellow in pulmonary and critical care medicine at Johns Hopkins University School of Medicine. In addition, he was a postdoctoral fellow in environmental health science at the Johns Hopkins University School of Hygiene and Public Health.

Deborah Schrag, M.D., is the chief of the Division of Population Sciences at the Dana-Farber Cancer Institute and a professor of medicine at Harvard Medical School in Boston, Massachusetts. Dr. Schrag is a health services researcher and a gastrointestinal medical oncologist with a focus on colorectal cancer. Her research focuses on improving the quality, effectiveness, and cost-effectiveness of cancer care delivery. She leads the Harvard Program in Cancer Care Delivery Research, is the principal investigator of several multi-center trials, and leads efforts to develop data standards to characterize outcomes of cancer treatment at population scale. She has performed foundational work in patient-reported outcomes and building phenomic data standards to systematically measure outcomes from electronic health records. Dr. Schrag is an associate editor of the *Journal of the American Medical Association*, a fellow of the American Society of Clinical Oncology and a former board director, a member of the National Academies of Sciences, Engineering, and Medicine's National

Cancer Policy Forum, and an elected member of the American Association of Physicians.

Ya Chen Tina Shih, Ph.D., is a professor in the Department of Health Services Research and holds the Hubert L. and Olive Stringer Professorship for Cancer Treatment and Research at the University of Texas MD Anderson Cancer Center. She is also the chief of the Section of Cancer Economics and Policy in the Department of Health Services Research at the university. She applies methods of health economics, health services research, and pharmacoeconomics in medical research, in particular, cancer research. She studies the diffusion of new medical technologies among patients, providers, and geographic areas; examines the impact of new technologies on the outcomes and costs of cancer care; and conducts methodological research on the analysis of medical cost data. She is the associate editor of the *Journal of the National Cancer Institute* and is on the editorial boards of *Value in Health*, *PharmacoEconomics*, and *JCO: Oncology Practice*. She is a member of the American Cancer Society guidelines development workgroup and was a member of the National Cancer Policy Forum at the National Academies of Sciences, Engineering, and Medicine. She received her Ph.D. in economics from Stanford University.

Kenneth Silverman, M.S., is the director of packaging technology in global technical operations at AstraZeneca. He manages a team of engineers responsible for commercializing innovative, standardized, sustainable commercial package systems for protein-based therapeutics, including monoclonal antibodies, antibody drug conjugates, mRNA, DNA, enzymes, gene therapy, and cell therapy. He entered biopharmaceutical research and development over two decades ago as a lab manager for developing packaging systems for new protein-based therapeutics at Schering–Plough. He moved into medical device research and development at Merck Research Laboratories focusing on design control methodologies to assess and mitigate risk and ensure optimal device packaging system development from prototype to a commercially scalable device design for biologics. In 2012 he moved out of research and development into technical operations at Bristol-Myers Squibb, where he developed packaging, scaled up manufacturing, and commercially launched immuno-oncology therapies including Opdivo, Yervoy, and Empliciti. At Bristol-Myers Squibb, he advanced from principal engineer to associate director where he harmonized and standardized Bristol-Myers Squibb's global packaging footprint for biologics. Mr. Silverman Joined AstraZeneca in January 2018 and he is responsible for all biological packaging from late-stage new molecular entities to commercialized products including Imfinzi, Fasenra, and Lumoxiti. He is currently responsible for ensuring an uninterrupted supply of protein-based therapeutics with a focus on optimal package design, excellence in manufacturing, harmonization, interchangeability, sustainability, and simplicity. He is the single patent holder for a senior-friendly single-dose dispensing package (WO2009149267). He received his master's degree and bachelor of science degree in packaging science from the Rochester Institute of Technology.

Holly Taylor, Ph.D., M.P.H., is a research bioethicist in the Department of Bioethics in the Clinical Center at the National Institutes of Health. She is a social scientist by training and has 20 years of experience conducting quantitative and qualitative research in the field of research ethics. Until 2019 she was an associate professor in the Department of Health Policy and Management at the Johns Hopkins Bloomberg School of Public Health and core faculty of the Berman Institute of Bioethics. She has served on institutional review boards at the Johns Hopkins Bloomberg School of Public Health and the Johns Hopkins University School of Medicine as well as in the government and private sector. Her primary interests are research ethics, local implementation of federal policy relevant to human subject research, and qualitative research methods. She earned a Ph.D. in bioethics and health policy from the Department of Health Policy and Management and Johns Hopkins Bloomberg School of Public Health, an M.P.H. from the University of Michigan School of Public Health, and a B.A. in human biology from Stanford University.

Jonathan Watanabe, Pharm.D., Ph.D., is a professor of clinical pharmacy and the associate dean of assessment and quality at the University of California (UC), Irvine, School of Pharmacy and Pharmaceutical Sciences. He was previously an associate professor of clinical pharmacy in the Skaggs School of Pharmacy and Pharmaceutical Sciences at UC San Diego. His research at UC San Diego focuses on pharmaceutical economic policy and health outcomes to improve health at the population level by examining how to improve medication-related health outcomes, particularly for the elderly and underserved populations. He served as an investigator and a fellowship director for the San Diego Geriatrics Workforce Enhancement Program. He is a clinical consultant for the Program of All-Inclusive Care for the Elderly (PACE) Clinic in San Diego, California. He was the inaugural recipient of the University of Washington/Allergan Global Health Economics and Outcomes Research Fellowship. He serves the California state legislature as a faculty content expert for the California Health Benefits Review Program and was a member of the advisory group on pain assessment and management standards for long-term care organizations for The Joint Commission. He is a board-certified geriatric pharmacist. He received a B.S. in zoology from the University of Washington, a Pharm.D. from the University of Southern California, and an M.S. and a Ph.D. from the University of Washington. He was the recipient of the third National Academy of Medicine (NAM) fellowship in pharmacy and is currently an inaugural scholar in the NAM Emerging Leaders in Health and Medicine program.

Alastair Wood, M.B., Ch.B., is an emeritus professor of medicine and an emeritus professor of pharmacology at Vanderbilt University. Previously he was the assistant vice chancellor for clinical research and the associate dean of Vanderbilt Medical School. He has served as a professor of medicine and pharmacology at Weill Cornell Medical College in New York and has served on a number of editorial boards. He was a member of the *New England Journal of Medicine* editorial board, served as the drug therapy editor of the *New England Journal of Medicine,* and was on the editorial board of the *British Journal of Clinical Pharmacology* and *The Scientist.* He has previously served on the editorial boards of *Clinical Pharmacology and Therapeutics* and *Biopharmaceutics and Drug Disposition.* He authored the chapter in *Harrison's Principles of Internal Medicine* on adverse drug reactions from the 9th through the 15th edition. He received his medical degree from St Andrews University and Dundee Medical School in Scotland. He is a member of the National Academy of Medicine.

K. Robin Yabroff, Ph.D., is an epidemiologist and the senior scientific director of health services research at the American Cancer Society. She also serves as an adjunct associate professor in the Department of Medicine at Johns Hopkins University and an adjunct professor in the Department of Health Policy and Management in the Rollins School of Public Health at Emory University. Prior to joining the Surveillance and Health Services Research Program at the American Cancer Society, she held positions within the Office of Health Policy of the Assistant Secretary for Planning and Evaluation in the U.S. Department of Health and Human Services, in the Health Services and Economics Branch of the National Cancer Institute, and in the faculty of the Lombardi Cancer Center at Georgetown University. She is an associate editor for the *Journal of the National Cancer Institute,* a founding member of the editorial board of the *Journal of Cancer Survivorship,* and a member of the editorial board of the *Journal of Oncology Practice.* She served as a guest editor for the *Medical Care* journal supplement, Health Care Costing: Data, Methods, Future Directions, and the *Journal of the National Cancer Institute* journal supplement Comparing Cancer Care and Economic Outcomes Across Health Systems: Challenges and Opportunities. She holds an M.B.A. from the University of Rochester and her Ph.D. in epidemiology from the Johns Hopkins Bloomberg School of Public Health.

Since the release of this report, it was determined that two members of the committee had financial conflicts of interest during the course of the study that had not been fully disclosed.

Dr. Anupum Jena provided compensated expert litigation consulting services in 2020 and 2021 to pharmaceutical companies including Merck, Genentech, Sanofi-Aventis, Janssen, and others through his affiliation with Analysis Group. Although these cases did not directly involve discarded drugs, because the recommendations of the study could be viewed as having a direct impact on the financial interests of some of these companies, the National Academies have concluded that Dr. Jena had a financial conflict of interest during the course of the study.

Dr. Gary Lyman made invited presentations in 2020 regarding the American Society of Clinical Oncology (ASCO) clinical practice guidelines for complications of cancer chemotherapy, the development of clinical pathways in oncology, and the work of the ASCO taskforce on biosimilars for which he received compensation from Jazz Pharmaceuticals, Merck Sharp & Dohme, Partner Therapeutics, Sandoz, and Seagen. Although the topics of these presentations were not directly related to the specific questions addressed by the committee, because the recommendations of the study could be viewed as having a direct impact on the financial interests of some of these companies, the National Academies have concluded that Dr. Lyman had a financial conflict of interest during the course of the study.

STAFF

Francis Kwadwo Amankwah, M.P.H., is a program officer in the Health and Medicine Division of the National Academies of Sciences, Engineering, and Medicine. He is the project lead on the National Academies study on the implications of discarded drugs resulting from weight-based dosing of medications contained in single-dose vials. He recently led a workshop that examined the role of the National Institutes of Health in drug development innovation and its impact on patient access. His portfolio of work at the National Academies has included providing research and analytical support in the development of the consensus study reports *Guiding Cancer Control: A Path to Transformation*; *Making Medicines Affordable: A National Imperative*; *Preventing Bullying Through Science, Policy, and Practice*; and *Promoting the Educational Success of Children and Youth Learning English: Promising Futures*. For his work at the National Academies, he has received the Mount Everest and the Fineberg Impact staff achievement awards from the Health and Medicine Division. He earned his M.P.H. and a graduate certificate in global planning and international development from Virginia Tech. He was raised in Ghana and earned his B.S. in agricultural science from the Kwame Nkrumah University of Science and Technology.

Alexandra (Allie) Andrada, M.A., is an associate program officer in the Health and Medicine Division of the National Academies of Sciences, Engineering, and Medicine, working on the consensus study on the implication of discarded weight-based drugs. Prior to joining the National Academies, she served as a lead research scientist supporting the Defense Health Board and the Defense Health Agency by producing technical reports on various public health topics affecting the military, such as child abuse and neglect and low-volume, high-risk surgical procedures throughout the Military Health System. She also has experience in survey research and design, program evaluation, guiding cognitive interviews, and conducting quantitative analyses focusing on military families, behavioral health, and at-risk youth. She earned her M.A. in experimental/biological psychology with a concentration in neuropsychology from American University and her B.S. in psychology and criminal justice from Virginia Commonwealth University.

Annalee Gonzales is an administrative assistant with the Board on Health Care Services and the National Cancer Policy Forum at the National Academies of Sciences, Engineering, and Medicine. She previously served as a senior program assistant for two reports from the National Academies on peer victimization and bullying and on fostering school success for English and dual-language learners. Prior to joining the National Academies she worked as an editorial and administrative coordinator at the National Association for Bilingual Education. She earned her B.A. in communication from Trinity University.

Tracy A. Lustig, D.P.M., M.P.H., is a senior program officer with the Health and Medicine Division of the National Academies of Sciences, Engineering, and Medicine. Dr. Lustig was trained in podiatric medicine and surgery and spent several years in private practice. In 1999 she was awarded a congressional fellowship with the American Association for the Advancement of Science and spent 1 year working in the office of Ron Wyden of the U.S. Senate. She joined the National Academies in 2004. Much of her work has focused on the health care workforce and the aging of the U.S. population. She was the study director for consensus studies on the geriatrics workforce, oral health, ovarian cancer research, and social isolation and loneliness in older adults. She also directed workshops on the allied health workforce, the use of telehealth to serve rural populations, assistive technologies, hearing loss, and artificial intelligence. In 2009 she staffed a National Academies–wide initiative on the "Grand Challenges of an Aging Society" and subsequently helped to launch the Forum on Aging, Disability, and Independence, which she currently directs. She has a doctor of podiatric medicine degree from Temple University and an M.P.H. with a concentration in health policy from The George Washington University.

Sharyl J. Nass, Ph.D., serves as the senior director of the Board on Health Care Services and the director of the National Cancer Policy Forum at the National Academies of Sciences, Engineering, and Medicine. The National Academies provide independent, objective analysis and advice to the nation to solve complex problems and inform public policy decisions related to science, technology, and medicine. To enable the best possible care for all patients, the board undertakes scholarly analysis of the organization, financing, effectiveness, workforce, and delivery of health care, with emphasis on quality, cost, and accessibility. The cancer forum examines policy issues pertaining to the entire continuum of cancer research and care. For two decades, Dr. Nass has worked on a broad range of health and science policy topics that include the quality and safety of health care and clinical trials, developing technologies for precision medicine, and strategies for large-scale biomedical science. She has a Ph.D. in cell biology from Georgetown University and undertook postdoctoral training at the Johns Hopkins University School of Medicine as well as a research fellowship at the Max Planck Institute in Germany. She also holds a B.S. and an M.S. from the University of Wisconsin–Madison. She has been the recipient of the Cecil Medal for Excellence in Health Policy Research, a distinguished service award from the National Academies, and the Institute of Medicine staff team achievement award (as team leader).

Appendix E

Disclosure of Unavoidable Conflicts of Interest

The conflict of interest policy of the National Academies of Sciences, Engineering, and Medicine (http://www.nationalacademies.org/coi) prohibits the appointment of an individual to a committee authoring a Consensus Study Report if the individual has a conflict of interest that is relevant to the task to be performed. An exception to this prohibition is permitted if the National Academies determines that the conflict is unavoidable and the conflict is publicly disclosed. A determination of a conflict of interest for an individual is not an assessment of that individual's actual behavior or character or ability to act objectively despite the conflicting interest.

Dr. Harold Paz has a conflict of interest in relation to his service on the Committee on Implications of Discarded Weight-Based Drugs because he currently owns shares of stock of United Surgical Partners International and CVS Health. Dr. Paz received financial remuneration from CVS Health through the end of May 2020. Also, he receives financial remuneration for his service on the United Surgical Partners International advisory board.

Mr. Kenneth Silverman has a conflict of interest in relation to his service on the Committee on Implications of Discarded Weight-Based Drugs because he is currently employed by a pharmaceutical manufacturer, AstraZeneca, as the director of packaging technology, global technical operations. Also, Mr. Silverman is the single patent holder for a senior-friendly single-dose dispensing package (WO2009149267).

In each case, the National Academies determined that the experience and expertise of the individual was needed for the committee to accomplish the task for which it had been established. The National Academies could not find other available individuals with the equivalent experience and expertise who do not have a conflict of interest. Therefore, the National Academies concluded that the conflict was unavoidable and publicly disclosed it through the National Academies Projects and Activities Repository (https://www8.nationalacademies.org/pa/projectview.aspx?key=51747).